Newborn Screening for Cystic Fibrosis

Newborn Screening for Cystic Fibrosis

Editors

Jürg Barben
Kevin W. Southern

MDPI • Basel • Beijing • Wuhan • Barcelona • Belgrade • Manchester • Tokyo • Cluj • Tianjin

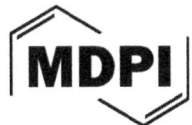

Editors
Jürg Barben
Children's Hospital of Eastern Switzerland
St. Gallen
Switzerland

Kevin W. Southern
University of Liverpool
Liverpool
United Kingdom

Editorial Office
MDPI
St. Alban-Anlage 66
4052 Basel, Switzerland

This is a reprint of articles from the Special Issue published online in the open access journal *International Journal of Neonatal Screening* (ISSN 2409-515X) (available at: https://www.mdpi.com/journal/IJNS/special_issues/cf).

For citation purposes, cite each article independently as indicated on the article page online and as indicated below:

LastName, A.A.; LastName, B.B.; LastName, C.C. Article Title. *Journal Name* **Year**, *Article Number*, Page Range.

ISBN 978-3-03936-990-4 (Hbk)
ISBN 978-3-03936-991-1 (PDF)

Cover image courtesy of Kevin Southern.

© 2020 by the authors. Articles in this book are Open Access and distributed under the Creative Commons Attribution (CC BY) license, which allows users to download, copy and build upon published articles, as long as the author and publisher are properly credited, which ensures maximum dissemination and a wider impact of our publications.

The book as a whole is distributed by MDPI under the terms and conditions of the Creative Commons license CC BY-NC-ND.

Contents

About the Editors . . . . **vii**

Jürg Barben and Kevin W. Southern
Why Do We Screen Newborn Infants for Cystic Fibrosis?
Reprinted from: *Int. J. Neonatal Screen.* 2020, 6, 56, doi:10.3390/ijns6030056 1

Carlo Castellani
Newborn Screening for Cystic Fibrosis: Over the Hump, Still Need to Fine-Tune It
Reprinted from: *Int. J. Neonatal Screen.* 2020, 6, 57, doi:10.3390/ijns6030057 5

Georges Travert, Mary Heeley and Anthony Heeley
History of Newborn Screening for Cystic Fibrosis—The Early Years
Reprinted from: *Int. J. Neonatal Screen.* 2020, 6, 8, doi:10.3390/ijns6010008 7

Lutz Naehrlich
The Changing Face of Cystic Fibrosis and Its Implications for Screening
Reprinted from: *Int. J. Neonatal Screen.* 2020, 6, 54, doi:10.3390/ijns6030054 15

Natasha Heather and Dianne Webster
It All Depends What You Count—The Importance of Definitions in Evaluation of CF Screening Performance
Reprinted from: *Int. J. Neonatal Screen.* 2020, 6, 47, doi:10.3390/ijns6020047 23

Virginie Scotet, Hector Gutierrez and Philip M. Farrell
Newborn Screening for CF across the Globe—*Where Is It Worthwhile*?
Reprinted from: *Int. J. Neonatal Screen.* 2020, 6, 18, doi:10.3390/ijns6010018 29

Rachael E. Armstrong, Lucy Frith, Fiona M. Ulph and Kevin W. Southern
Constructing a Bioethical Framework to Evaluate and Optimise Newborn Bloodspot Screening for Cystic Fibrosis
Reprinted from: *Int. J. Neonatal Screen.* 2020, 6, 40, doi:10.3390/ijns6020040 47

Olaf Sommerburg and Jutta Hammermann
Pancreatitis-Associated Protein in Neonatal Screening for Cystic Fibrosis: Strengths and Weaknesses
Reprinted from: *Int. J. Neonatal Screen.* 2020, 6, 28, doi:10.3390/ijns6020028 61

Anne Bergougnoux, Maureen Lopez and Emmanuelle Girodon
The Role of Extended *CFTR* Gene Sequencing in Newborn Screening for Cystic Fibrosis
Reprinted from: *Int. J. Neonatal Screen.* 2020, 6, 23, doi:10.3390/ijns6010023 75

Anne Munck
Inconclusive Diagnosis after Newborn Screening for Cystic Fibrosis
Reprinted from: *Int. J. Neonatal Screen.* 2020, 6, 19, doi:10.3390/ijns6010019 91

Jürg Barben and Jane Chudleigh
Processing Newborn Bloodspot Screening Results for CF
Reprinted from: *Int. J. Neonatal Screen.* 2020, 6, 25, doi:10.3390/ijns6020025 99

Jane Chudleigh and Holly Chinnery
Psychological Impact of NBS for CF
Reprinted from: *Int. J. Neonatal Screen.* 2020, 6, 27, doi:10.3390/ijns6020027 109

About the Editors

Jürg Barben is Professor of Pediatric Pulmonology at the University of Basel and heads the Department of Pediatric Pulmonology & Allergology and the CF Center at the Children's Hospital of Eastern Switzerland in St. Gallen. He has been doing research in the field of cystic fibrosis for many years, especially in the field of diagnostics (sweat test and newborn screening), and established the Newborn Screening (NBS) Programme for CF in Switzerland in 2011. He was President of the Swiss Working Group for CF for eight years until 2014 and has been the Chair of the CF Group of the European Respiratory Society (ERS) since 2017. Since 2019, he has coordinated the Newborn Screening Working Group (NSWG) of the European CF Society (ECFS).

Kevin W. Southern is Professor of Pediatric Pulmonology at the University of Liverpool and works at the Alder Hey Children's Hospital. He is the Director of a network responsible for the care of over 300 children with CF in the North West of England. In 2007, he helped establish the national UK NBS Programme for CF, and he now chairs the national Board overseeing this programme. Until 2019, he had been the Leader of the ECFS NSWG for more than ten years. He is an Editor for the International Cochrane Review Group and he has written and contributed to many systematic reviews. His research is focused on translating evidence into practice, and he has published over 100 peer-reviewed articles on CF. He is the joint editor of the textbook *"Early CF Years"*, sponsored by the ECFS, and he was an elected member of the ECFS Board for seven years until 2019.

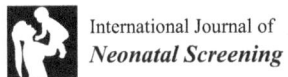

International Journal of
Neonatal Screening

Editorial

Why Do We Screen Newborn Infants for Cystic Fibrosis?

Jürg Barben [1],* and Kevin W. Southern [2],*

1. Division of Paediatric Pulmonology & CF Centre, Children's Hospital of Eastern Switzerland, 9006 St. Gallen, Switzerland
2. Department of Women's and Children's Health, University of Liverpool, Alder Hey Children's Hospital NHS Foundation Trust, Liverpool L12 2AP, UK
* Correspondence: Juerg.Barben@kispisg.ch (J.B.); kwsouth@liverpool.ac.uk (K.W.S.)

Received: 6 July 2020; Accepted: 6 July 2020; Published: 8 July 2020

The introduction and widespread implementation of newborn bloodspot screening (NBS) for cystic fibrosis (CF) has offered earlier diagnosis and better outcomes for children with CF in many countries of the world. It represents a paradigm shift in the diagnostic pathway for these families. In contrast to a clinical diagnosis, infants are now referred for diagnostic testing after a positive NBS result and, apart from a small proportion who present with bowel obstruction (meconium ileus), CF infants have no or only minimal clinical manifestation of the disease in the early days of life. Clinical symptoms can appear over the first few weeks, for example, insufficient weight gain, fatty stools or salt loss syndrome, but are often insidious and difficult to recognise.

The introduction of NBS has enabled the provision of early appropriate treatment (pancreatic enzyme replacement therapy, fat-soluble vitamins, salt supplementation and antibiotics) to prevent manifestations of the disease. In the near future, early diagnosis will facilitate the prompt use of new cystic fibrosis transmembrane conductance regulator (CFTR) modulator therapies that correct the basic underlying molecular defect.

NBS for CF has been a global success but continues to raise questions with many varied approaches and the development of new technologies, in particular the ability to undertake extensive gene examination. It is still valid to ask many questions:

- What is the best protocol to achieve high sensitivity and specificity?
- Should extensive genetic analysis be part of this algorithm, which enables the identification of many more *CFTR* variants?
- How to evaluate and manage inconclusive cases with a borderline sweat test or CFTR variants with unclear clinical relevance?
- What is the optimal approach to inform and counsel the parents about the NBS results and inconclusive findings?

These questions are not easy to answer and require a balanced solution that reflects the local health care system and may appropriately result in different answers around the globe.

The aim of this series of articles was to compile the current state of knowledge on NBS for CF and the questions arising from it. Using the framework of the network of the Newborn Screening Working Group (NSWG) of the European CF Society (ECFS), we approached colleagues from all over the world to submit articles for peer review. On the initiative of the *International Journal of Newborn Screening* (IJNS), the opportunity arose to realize this project, and we would like to take this opportunity to thank the authors for their excellent contributions and the IJNS for their support and cooperation. We feel the resulting series of articles provides a state-of-the-art evaluation of the current status of NBS for CF and provides much insight into the questions above and a path to improve quality across the globe.

The history of newborn bloodspot screening for CF is recorded by Georges Travert and Mary and Anthony Heeley, all of whom played an important role in these early developments. They cover the early use of the immune-reactive trypsinogen (IRT) assay, the challenges they and others faced and how they were overcome [1].

Lutz Naehrlich describes how early diagnosis, multidisciplinary care and optimized and preventive treatments have improved the outlook for people with CF. From his position as Director of the European Registry, he is able to give a clear picture of the changing face of CF, and the direct impact of NBS on this landscape [2].

One of the major challenges in the field of NBS for CF has been the collection of robust and comparable data across countries and regions. New Zealand was the first country to establish NBS for CF and Natasha Heather and Dianne Webster are well placed to reflect on the importance and challenges of collecting the correct metrics [3]. They highlight the critical importance of this if the quality of this public health initiative is to improve.

Virginie Scotet, Hector Gutierrez and Philip M. Farrell give an overview about the current situation of NBS for CF across the globe [4]. Each region has typically undertaken CF NBS after analysis of the advantages, costs and challenges, particularly regarding the relationship of benefits to risks. The review describes the lessons learned from the journey toward universal screening wherever CF is prevalent and an analytical framework for application in those undecided regions.

This complements the next article, in which Rachel Armstrong, Lucy Frith, Fiona Ulph and Kevin Southern consider NBS for CF from a bioethical perspective [5]. They report in detail all possible outcomes from NBS for CF and place these in an ethical framework. Placing these in the context of the genetic profile of the population screened, the geography of the region and the healthcare resources available, they propose an approach engaging with stakeholders to determine the best protocol for a region.

Olaf Sommerburg and Jutta Hammermann describe in their review the strengths and weaknesses of pancreatitis-associated protein (PAP) in the algorithm of NBS for CF [6]. This biochemical test has emerged as an adjunct to IRT measurement, but the relationship is complex and is reviewed in detail by these authors who have considerable experience through implementing this assay as part of the protocol in Germany.

Anne Bergougnoux, Maureen Lopez and Emmanuelle Girodon give a summary of the role of DNA analysis in the CF screening programme. Their work in the national French laboratory gives them a unique insight into the challenges of incorporating genetic testing, especially extended gene analysis (EGA) [7].

A consequence of NBS for CF is the identification of infants with a positive screening test but an inconclusive diagnostic testing. Anne Munck led the European consensus exercise to better define the evaluation and management of these infants, in addition to leading the French research project that monitored outcomes. She places these results in the context of other work from around the globe [8].

The processing of a positive NBS result for CF not only consists of the screening part in the laboratory but also the interface between the family and healthcare, and ultimately the CF team. This is a complex process reviewed by Jürg Barben and Jane Chudleigh, both of whom have undertaken extensive research projects examining these issues [9]. It is clear that this is an area that needs considerable improvement across the globe and the authors review evidence of good practice and propose a roadmap to improve the quality of this difficult process.

Consistent with the article above is a detailed review of the psychological impact of NBS for CF by Jane Chudleigh and Holly Chinnery [10]. A better understanding of the journey that the families of infants with a positive NBS result go on enables CF teams to predict and ameliorate unnecessary distress.

Again we thank all the authors; there is much to celebrate in the field of NBS for CF, but clearly still work to do, and this experienced faculty of authors has provided a series of state-of-the-art articles to help achieve that goal. In addition, we would like to thank the 19 experts who provided high-quality peer review (sometimes twice) for this series. We were extremely grateful for their comprehensive and timely contributions, which were important for the overall quality of the series.

Funding: This research received no external funding.

Conflicts of Interest: The authors declare no conflict of interest.

References

1. Travert, G.; Heeley, M.; Heeley, A. History of Newborn Screening for Cystic Fibrosis—The Early Years. *Int. J. Neonatal Screen.* **2020**, *6*, 8. [CrossRef]
2. Naehrlich, L. The Changing Face of Cystic Fibrosis and Its Implications for Screening. *Int. J. Neonatal Screen.* **2020**, *6*, 54. [CrossRef]
3. Heather, N.; Webster, D. It All Depends What You Count—The Importance of Definitions in Evaluation of CF Screening Performance. *Int. J. Neonatal Screen.* **2020**, *6*, 47. [CrossRef]
4. Scotet, V.; Gutierrez, H.; Farrell, P.M. Newborn Screening for CF across the Globe—*Where Is It Worthwhile*? *Int. J. Neonatal Screen.* **2020**, *6*, 18. [CrossRef]
5. Armstrong, R.E.; Frith, L.; Ulph, F.M.; Southern, K.W. Constructing a Bioethical Framework to Evaluate and Optimise Newborn Bloodspot Screening for Cystic Fibrosis. *Int. J. Neonatal Screen.* **2020**, *6*, 40. [CrossRef]
6. Sommerburg, O.; Hammermann, J. Pancreatitis-Associated Protein in Neonatal Screening for Cystic Fibrosis: Strengths and Weaknesses. *Int. J. Neonatal Screen.* **2020**, *6*, 28. [CrossRef]
7. Bergougnoux, A.; Lopez, M.; Girodon, E. The Role of Extended *CFTR* Gene Sequencing in Newborn Screening for Cystic Fibrosis. *Int. J. Neonatal Screen.* **2020**, *6*, 23. [CrossRef]
8. Munck, A. Inconclusive Diagnosis after Newborn Screening for Cystic Fibrosis. *Int. J. Neonatal Screen.* **2020**, *6*, 19. [CrossRef]
9. Barben, J.; Chudleigh, J. Processing Newborn Bloodspot Screening Results for CF. *Int. J. Neonatal Screen.* **2020**, *6*, 25. [CrossRef]
10. Chudleigh, J.; Chinnery, H. Psychological Impact of NBS for CF. *Int. J. Neonatal Screen.* **2020**, *6*, 27. [CrossRef]

© 2020 by the authors. Licensee MDPI, Basel, Switzerland. This article is an open access article distributed under the terms and conditions of the Creative Commons Attribution (CC BY) license (http://creativecommons.org/licenses/by/4.0/).

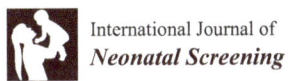

Editorial

Newborn Screening for Cystic Fibrosis: Over the Hump, Still Need to Fine-Tune It

Carlo Castellani

Cystic Fibrosis Center, IRCCS Istituto Giannina Gaslini, 16147 Genoa, Italy; carlocastellani@gaslini.org

Received: 6 July 2020; Accepted: 6 July 2020; Published: 9 July 2020

Today, newborn screening (NBS) is considered an essential component in the standards of care for cystic fibrosis (CF) [1] and, to cite a well-known paper, "a basic human right" [2]. This has not always been the case and, in a not too remote past, the appropriateness of screening neonates for CF was much debated. In those days, NBS had been implemented in very few areas, and was more often a research project than an established health program. Decision-makers were waiting for proof that early diagnosis was an opportunity to modify the natural history of CF. That sort of evidence was not easy to collect for a disease characterized by wide genotype and phenotype diversity and a long term clinical evolution, and the very few randomized controlled trials struggled to prove the point [3,4]. Over time, direct and circumstantial evidence in favour of the benefits of CF NBS accumulated [5] and its practice progressively extended to most countries with predominantly Caucasian populations. A further acceleration came from the emergence of small molecules targeting the defective CF transmembrane regulator (CFTR) protein. These compounds, although only partially rescuing CFTR function and not yet available to all patients or licensed for use in the first months of life, might prevent or greatly delay the development of disease manifestations if started at the youngest possible age.

Currently, the vast majority of newborns in North America and Europe, and a growing number in South America, are screened for CF. The expansion phase of CF NBS has probably reached its summit and is gradually slowing down. Nevertheless, it remains crucial and urgent to support the implementation of NBS in countries where CF shows a significant prevalence, that can capitalize on the competence accumulated elsewhere and avoid the errors made by those who preceded them.

It is also critical to make the actual screening strategies as effective and as efficient as possible. Guidelines are available [1,6] and provide direction, but advice can be challenging to implement in distinct genetic, logistic and strategic environments. There is no model that fits all the variables that characterize different areas, and each protocol has to be customized for local needs. Sharing expertise and learning from others' experience may help to tune up the many components of each screening strategy and, on a personal level, to improve the daily practice of lab workers, CF doctors and nurses.

The articles in this issue of the *International Journal of Neonatal Screening* offer a state-of-the-art scrutiny of several aspects of CF NBS and contribute to the debate on some old but still burning questions. Some of them are connected with the inclusion of molecular genetics in CF NBS, now used in most protocols for its potential to improve specificity and the timing of the screening procedures. Technological improvements have made it possible and affordable to tailor mutation panels to local requirements but have also offered the option to move to non-mutation-specific analysis. Next generation sequencing allows for the fast identification of all exome variations, with a sensitivity far superior to any pre-set mutation kit. This does constitute an asset in populations with extreme genetic variability, but it may uncover information whose clinical significance is difficult or even impossible to interpret.

CF screening positive, inconclusive diagnosis (CFSPID), also known as CFTR related metabolic syndrome (CRMS), in infants may be detected by NBS strategies that do not include genetic analysis, but many more are found if DNA in IRT-positive samples is sequenced. We are now witnessing a situation somewhat similar to that already experienced with the identification of carriers through

CF NBS. This was and is still seen with favour by some, who consider it an opportunity to explore the extended family of the carrier neonate and find couples at high risk of having children with CF, whereas most consider it an undesirable effect of the screening procedure. Similarly, the identification of CFSPID/CRMS infants may be regarded as the occasion for monitoring children who might, over time evolve CF, or as a distressing intrusion in the life of parents whose child may develop late and mild, or even no symptoms at all. None of these considerations can be dismissed as incorrect, but if we agree that the purpose of CF NBS is the early finding of infants with a severe disease and, thereby, to be able to offer prompt treatment, carrier and CFSPID/CRMS children are probably to be considered more an unwanted consequence than a collateral benefit of CF NBS. Concerns about the inclusion of molecular analysis in CF NBS have driven the search for non-genetic assays that could compensate for the limited specificity of IRT. So far, the only option appears to be the pancreatitis associated protein (PAP), which cannot substitute IRT but rather complements it in elaborate screening algorithms.

CF NBS has reached a mature stage of its development and is widely considered an indispensable part of CF care. The debate has now shifted from usefulness to optimization and focused on the containment and management of collateral outcomes, reliable data collection in specific registries and quality monitoring. It is important to keep the dialogue alive among stakeholders, and in this regard this Special Issue is a valuable and timely resource.

Funding: This research received no external funding.

Conflicts of Interest: The author declares no conflict of interest.

References

1. Castellani, C.; Duff, A.J.; Bell, S.C.; Heijerman, H.G.; Munck, A.; Ratjen, F.; Sermet-Gaudelus, I.; Southern, K.W.; Barben, J.; Flume, P.A.; et al. ECFS best practice guidelines: The 2018 revision. *J. Cyst. Fibros.* **2018**, *17*, 153–178. [CrossRef] [PubMed]
2. Farrell, P.M. Is newborn screening for cystic fibrosis a basic human right? *J. Cyst. Fibros.* **2008**, *7*, 262–265. [CrossRef] [PubMed]
3. Farrell, P.M.; Kosorok, M.R.; Laxova, A.; Shen, G.; Koscik, R.E.; Bruns, W.T.; Splaingard, M.; Mischler, E.H. Nutritional benefits of neonatal screening for cystic fibrosis. *N. Engl. J. Med.* **1997**, *337*, 963–969. [CrossRef] [PubMed]
4. Chatfield, S.; Owen, G.; Ryley, H.C.; Williams, J.; Alfaham, M.; Goodchild, M.C.; Weller, P. Neonatal screening for cystic fibrosis in Wales and the West Midlands: Clinical assessment after five years of screening. *Arch. Dis. Child.* **1991**, *66*, 29–33. [CrossRef] [PubMed]
5. Castellani, C.; Massie, J.; Sontag, M.; Southern, K.W. Newborn screening for cystic fibrosis. *Lancet Respir. Med.* **2016**, *4*, 653–661. [CrossRef]
6. Castellani, C.; Southern, K.W.; Brownlee, K.; Roelse, J.D.; Duff, A.; Farrell, M.; Mehta, A.; Munck, A.; Pollitt, R.; Sermet-Gaudelus, I.; et al. European best practice guidelines for cystic fibrosis neonatal screening. *J. Cyst. Fibros.* **2009**, *8*, 153–173. [CrossRef] [PubMed]

© 2020 by the author. Licensee MDPI, Basel, Switzerland. This article is an open access article distributed under the terms and conditions of the Creative Commons Attribution (CC BY) license (http://creativecommons.org/licenses/by/4.0/).

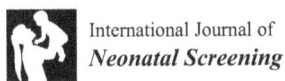

Review

History of Newborn Screening for Cystic Fibrosis—The Early Years

Georges Travert [1,2,*]**, Mary Heeley** [3] **and Anthony Heeley** [3]

1. University of Caen Normandy (UNICAEN), 14032 Caen, France
2. Caen University Hospital, 14040 Caen, France
3. East Anglian Biochemical Genetic Unit, Peterborough, UK
* Correspondence: georges.travert@wanadoo.fr

Received: 20 December 2019; Accepted: 28 January 2020; Published: 31 January 2020

Abstract: This review summarises the trajectory of neonatal screening strategies for the detection of cystic fibrosis (CF) using the measurement of Immunoreactive Trypsin (IRT) in dried blood spots (DBS) from 1979 until the beginning of the 21st century when newborn screening (NBS) programmes started to spread throughout many countries, using IRT measurement combined with a CF genotype analysis of DBS.

Keywords: newborn screening; immunoreactive trypsin(ogen); dried blood spot; radioimmunoassay; DNA

1. The Background

In the 1950s, Dr. Harry Shwachman, paediatrician at Boston Children's Hospital, recognised that early diagnosis was an important factor underpinning the optimal outcome for cystic fibrosis (CF) patients, receiving both nutritional support and an aggressive treatment of lung infections [1]. However, at this time, no neonatal screening test had been described.

The first attempts at newborn screening (NBS) for CF were performed in the 1970s [2] and were based on a semi quantitative measurement of the albumin content in meconium (BM test). However, elevated meconium albumin levels are a consequence of exocrine pancreatic insufficiency, and pancreatic sufficient CF neonates could not be detected (false negatives). The test also had a very high false positive rate, especially among preterm newborns. Due to its lack of specificity and sensitivity, screening trials with this test were not widely implemented; the exception being where the meconium specimens could be delivered directly from the maternity ward to a laboratory, usually closely associated with a CF clinical centre, where more elaborate testing could take place [3].

The detection of faecal tryptic activity using artificial peptide substrates was next in line for promotion as a potential screening test [4]. Although this eliminated some of the problems associated with meconium testing, the inability to detect pancreatic sufficient neonates would remain a problem. However, two contemporary developments brought these lines of investigation to an abrupt end, as described in the next section.

These and other issues of the period have been reviewed in detail elsewhere [5].

2. New Neonatal Screening Strategies Emerge

Newborn population screening for inherited/congenital diseases such as phenylketonuria (PKU) and congenital hypothyroidism (CHT) had been widely implemented by the late 1970s. Biochemical screening on this scale had been enabled through the innovative work of Robert Guthrie [6], who demonstrated that phenylalanine could be measured accurately in minute amounts of blood that were obtained by heel-prick, collected, and dried on absorbent paper (DBS). Dried blood had the advantage of conferring good stability of the analyte during transport to the laboratory and for later storage. Moreover, these specimens were shown to be suitable for the measurements of analytes in the nanogramme range, such as hormones, using the relatively new techniques of radio-immunoassay (RIA) as Jean Dussault in Quebec, Canada, demonstrated in 1975 with a NBS test for CHT [7].

The 1970s also saw a surge of interest in the role of exocrine proteins in gastrointestinal physiology and pathology. RIA based methods were developed, which were sufficiently sensitive to detect the extremely low concentrations present in the circulation. The pancreatic zymogen trypsinogen was one of these proteins, and the immediate clinical interest in this assay stemmed from its potential for use in the differential diagnosis of pancreatic disease. With this objective in mind, a number of commercial diagnostic companies had, by the late 1970s, developed RIA reagents for serum trypsin(ogen) (IRT) measurement. Although older CF patients with overt pancreatic insufficiency had subnormal serum IRT levels, surprisingly, IRT levels in early infancy were elevated irrespective of the patient's pancreatic functional status.

The collection of liquid blood and the separation of serum was a cumbersome procedure for neonatal biochemical screening purposes. Would the use of DBS, of proven reliability in other established NBS protocols, also be suitable for the measurement of IRT? The answer to this question came in 1979 from the laboratory of the Department of Paediatrics at Auckland (NZ) Medical School.

The short report by Crossley and co-workers [8] was notable not only for their development of an assay of sufficient sensitivity to measure IRT in dried blood spots but also that IRT was sufficiently stable in DBS form for it to be measurable after storage for many months or even several years. In this study, DBS IRT levels were able to clearly distinguish each of 23 CF neonates from two controls randomly selected in the same batch of Guthrie cards, despite the cards having been stored at room temperature for up to seven years. Therefore the repositories of DBS cards which had been used for PKU/CHT screening would be a valuable resource for the retrospective testing of newborn DBS of infants whose later diagnosis of CF had been established solely on clinical grounds, and in whom the clinical history would be well documented.

The importance of this seminal paper and the almost instantaneous confirmation of its findings in several laboratories cannot be overestimated. The retrospective DBS testing of historical CF infants clearly demonstrated that pre-symptomatic detection of the condition was possible. Even so, it remained unclear how efficient the DBS IRT assay would be in the prospective NBS setting. Additionally, there were aspects of the assay described by Crossley which were unsuitable for routine newborn population screening purposes, i.e., the size of blood spot required. This problem was quickly overcome [9], and the scene was set for prospective screening trials to begin.

3. The Two-Stage IRT Prospective Screening Trials (IRT–IRT) 1979–1989

In 1980, apart from the ongoing work in Auckland, there were two European screening laboratories that had the necessary technical and clinical infrastructure in place to incorporate IRT screening alongside their established PKU/CHT programmes. These laboratories were at Caen (France) and at Peterborough (UK), responsible for screening the newborn population of Normandy and East Anglia respectively. At the time, there were two commercially available serum IRT assays, both of which had been independently adapted for DBS IRT screening in these French and UK laboratories (Hoechst Behring Germany in Caen and Sorin Biomedica Italy in Peterborough).

For various complex technical reasons, particularly the lack of an internationally accepted standard preparation of human trypsin(ogen) the results obtained by these different RIAs would not be directly comparable. Each laboratory had to determine, for its own newborn population, the DBS IRT concentration that would provide an optimal screening cut-off.

Moreover, it appeared that hypertrypsinaemia occurs frequently in non-CF neonates during the first days of life, declining rapidly thereafter, whereas the hypertrypsinaemia of CF persists to some degree for several months. Thus, a few infants would have to be re-tested, preferably within the following 1–2 weeks, and, again, an optimal screening cut-off would have to be established for these older infants; those infants with a DBS IRT level above this cut-off level would be referred for diagnostic sweat testing and clinical assessment. Carrying out a sweat test on 4–6 week-old infants by the standard Gibson–Cooke procedure is difficult, cumbersome, and time consuming. In the early 1980s, an innovative sweat collection system was developed commercially, which greatly facilitated the testing of small infants in screening trials [10].

It was gratifying to find, as early as 1980, that the results obtained from the trials in Normandy and East Anglia with different assays were producing similar results, in particular, acceptable sensitivity and specificity for the detection of CF infants with low retest rates [11,12]. These preliminary results had, quite independently, in 1980 been disseminated to audiences of paediatricians and clinical biochemists known to be interested in this field of investigation (at Caen in October and London in November). Together with the ongoing work in Auckland (NZ), this led to a burgeoning of two-stage IRT screening trials in other countries, and, as a result, data began to accumulate more rapidly, particularly from those laboratories whose screening hinterland was more populous. Among the latter were New South Wales, Australia, Colorado, USA, and Alto Adige/Veneto, Italy. Initiating these trials, respectively, were Bridget Wilken (Sydney), Keith Hammond (Denver), and Gianni Mastella (Verona).

Two other trials with different objectives, namely to determine whether NBS was clinically effective, began in the mid-1980s. One of these, carried out in Wales/the West Midlands region (UK), elected to screen a large neonatal population for CF using the two-stage IRT method but only on alternate weeks. The other, undertaken in Wisconsin (USA), was an ambitious randomised control trial (RCT) in which half the results of the initial IRT screening test were randomly and anonymously blinded for a period of four years. In the active group, infants with positive IRT singleton test results were immediately referred for sweat testing and, if appropriate, clinical follow-up. However, these trials contributed little useful information regarding the efficacy of the IRT–IRT protocol because, in the case of the former, IRT testing was delayed for 3 weeks after the blood had been drawn, and because of the latter's aforementioned design [13,14].

As work progressed, it became necessary to convene meetings that would allow investigators to compare results in a timely manner. The first international round table discussions occurred in Peterborough in 1987, but, unfortunately, the sponsorship was insufficient to bring colleagues from the Antipodes. A more generous sponsorship, probably combined with the certain prospect of better food in Normandy, resulted in a widely attended conference with exceptionally fruitful discussions in Caen 1988. The issues addressed at these meetings were as follows: (1) IRT assay methodology. (2) The early nutritional status and respiratory function of the screened cohorts. (3) Optimal shared care between regional CF clinical centres and local paediatricians.

At that time, 9 laboratories from 7 countries had each screened in excess of 100,000 newborns, and although a majority of these had consistently achieved satisfactory test specificity and sensitivity, others had not. (The data were collected personally by G. Travert and reported in the proceedings of the International Conference: Mucoviscidose, Dépistage néonatal et Prise en charge précoce. Travert G (ed) Université de Caen 1988). The predictive value of a positive (IRT–IRT) test result ranged from 25%–86%, and a retest rate of the initially screened population varying between 0.3%–4.7%.

The reasons for these discrepancies could not be attributed to the type of RIA employed; nevertheless, these assays were inherently prone to sporadic technical error. Other likely confounding variables were the age of the initial and recall testing, age-related screening cut-offs, and the quality of DBS provided for screening, including the very high risk of contamination.

These and other issues relating to DBS IRT screening have been reviewed in more detail elsewhere [15,16]. Whatever the reasons for the variable results, the need for a within- and between-laboratory performance indicator had been unanimously advocated at a meeting convened in 1985 by G. Mastella in Verona, the organization of which was entrusted to the laboratories of Caen and Peterborough.

The IRT International Quality Assurance Scheme (IRTIQAS) began in 1987 with 16 laboratories from 6 countries. Dried blood spots were prepared from the blood of pancreatitis patients for elevated levels, and often laboratory staff for the control levels, and were distributed monthly. Because different reagents, techniques, and variations of the trypsin antigen were being used by the 16 participants, absolute values could not be compared. However, the scheme gave an indication of within- and between-assay performance and an assurance that laboratories had chosen the appropriate cut-off to distinguish a CF neonate with a minimum proportion of false positives. By 1990 there were 40 laboratories from 8 countries, a clear indication that the scheme was beneficial to laboratories in determining whether their CV and bias were consistent, at which point the manufacturer's agreed to contribute to the running costs. IRTIQAS was not ideal because the utilized DBS could not be obtained from CF newborns because the volume of blood needed was prohibitive. The lack of an international reference standard was a major drawback. The preliminary results emanating from this scheme were presented at the 1988 Caen Conference and in more detail at the later (1990) International Conference organized by K. Hammond at Estes Park, Colorado [17].

In order to eliminate the multistep, error prone, manual process and radiochemical facilities required for RIA, alternative immunoassay technologies were being introduced in diagnostic clinical chemistry. One of these utilised solid phase monoclonal antibodies, a second chemically labelled antibody and an enzyme linked signal amplification system. Assays of this type could be carried out in multi well antibody-coated microtitre plates with much enhanced and simplified sample throughput. Biochemists at the Queensland (Australia) neonatal screening laboratory in Brisbane had developed such an assay for DBS IRT [18] and a commercial version was launched at the 1988 Caen meeting. The latter generated much interest and some CF screening laboratories changed to this methodology abruptly, causing further confusion in the quest to determine which screening modality was most efficacious in the long term.

In the concluding address of this conference in Caen, the eminent geneticist Jean Frezal predicted that in the future genetic analysis would underpin neonatal screening for CF; a prescient prediction, because, within twelve months, the *CFTR* gene and its main mutation F508del had been described [19]. New horizons for newborn CF screening had been opened up.

4. IRT-DNA from 1990

Polymorphic alleles closely associated with the *CFTR* gene had been studied as a potential adjunct to IRT screening in the Normandy neonatal population with some success [20]. However, it was the elucidation of the *CFTR* gene structure and the identification of the F508del mutation with high prevalence in the CF population that provided the stimulus for virtually every major screening centre to embrace molecular genetic analytical techniques. Would the introduction of DNA analysis into the IRT–IRT protocol improve the screening test performance? Would it enable the recall second IRT test to be abolished? Results from some preliminary work were presented at the 1990 International meeting in Colorado. Somewhat surprisingly, the Adelaide laboratory of the South Australian Regional Programme, reported that they had already implemented IRT-DNA screening [21]. They had used a low cut-off (99th centile) on 5-day old infants followed by DBS DNA analysis for the mutations F508del and I507del, i.e., on 1% of the neonatal population. Whilst this protocol eliminated the recall of infants for further IRT testing, it could be cogently argued that it posed a number of problems: (a) sensitivity was limited to 94% (gene prevalence related), (b) all heterozygous infants had to be sweat tested and the parents of those infants with normal results (86%) were offered genetic counselling, (c) those infants that screened IRT positive, in whom either of these mutations was absent (94%), were reported "CF not indicated"; rather tenuously in view of the imposed limit of sensitivity. Most centres running IRT–IRT protocols had, by this time, achieved better sensitivity, fewer infants were recalled for sweat testing, and none of the dilemmas associated with the detection of heterozygotes arose.

At the same meeting, the Caen laboratory group reported investigations, both retrospective and prospective, with IRT-DNA (F508del) and their results showed convincingly that the introduction of DNA analysis, with its present limitations, would not be beneficial as an adjunct to IRT screening if the primary purpose was to maximise the detection of CF infants as soon as possible after birth.

Nevertheless, the South Australian work was important in demonstrating the feasibility of IRT-DNA neonatal screening in a routine setting. Its effectiveness would undoubtedly be improved with the inclusion of more CF mutations in the IRT-DNA protocol or in the inclusion of a third stage IRT-DNA-IRT [22].

An equally important contemporary finding from the Caen laboratory resulted from their investigation of F508del in the DBS of infants who had screened IRT negative but whose DBS IRT levels approached that of the designated discriminatory cut-off, i.e., the 99.5th centile. In the general French population, the prevalence of F508del healthy carriers is 2.5%–3%. Amongst neonates with low IRT levels, it was 0.5% but progressively reached 10–11% in healthy newborns with IRT levels just below or just above the cut-off [23,24]. The practical consequence of these findings was that any trend to lower the IRT cut-off value, in order to improve the screening sensitivity, would inevitably result in an increased detection rate of healthy carriers. Therefore, as early as 1990, potential problems associated with IRT-DNA screening had emerged. It would take another decade of more adjustments to decide how many of the increasing number of known *CFTR* gene mutations should be included in the screening process.

Unsurprisingly, many of these problems remain unresolved, including the category of screened patients now called CFSPID (CF Screen Positive, Inconclusive Diagnosis) in Europe and CFTR-related Metabolic Syndrome (CRMS) in the USA.

5. The Tide Turns 1998

At the instigation of the directors of the Normandy and New South Wales screening laboratories, a further meeting was convened in 1998 at Caen to mark the approaching second decade of newborn screening for CF and to take stock of progress over this period.

From their inception these International conferences had included the work of clinical psychologists, nutritionists, paediatricians, and CF nurses who had been involved with the individual trials [25,26]. Much had been learned about managing the social and ethical issues of CF screening, of the early natural history of the disease and its clinical management, all of which is covered in Jim Littlewood's comprehensive on-line historic review of CF [27].

Throughout the 1990s, more robust screening strategies had emerged by increasing the number of CFTR mutations in the DNA analysis. The DBS IRT assay had been substantially improved by the Wallac Co. in Finland, using more selective monoclonal antibodies and an extremely sensitive labelling technology with an analytical system that was already widely used in neonatal screening laboratories for the detection of CHT.

On balance, it seemed that the work that began in the early 1980s had been successfully concluded. The way forward would, in part, depend on local population demographics, ethical considerations, and the ability of health services to deliver optimal treatment for the condition. All that remained to further the case for CF newborn screening was incontrovertible evidence that early diagnosis and clinical intervention conferred significant future health benefits for these infants. That evidence was provided in the long-awaited results of the meticulous RCT conducted by Philip M. Farrell and colleagues in Wisconsin. While presenting these results in Caen in 1998, he concluded that "the burden of proof is now on those who argue against neonatal screening for CF" [26] (p.250).

This gauntlet was unlikely to be taken up by any serious contenders; the results of the Wisconsin trial were confirmation of what a whole generation of paediatricians caring for these patients already knew instinctively. It was also unlikely that any government public health service agency would ignore the evidence. Several NBS laboratories, as early as 1988, had secured health service funding from their respective state/regional public health authorities for the inclusion of CF in their NBS programme, which was justified by the short term clinical and diagnostic cost benefits gained. Before commissioning new public health screening services, national government agencies would normally seek stakeholder consensus for the best practice guidelines; the inclusion of molecular genetic analysis in the current CF NBS protocol presented a novel and more complex issue than had hitherto arisen in NBS commissioning.

Unsurprisingly, the time taken to introduce CF NBS at a national level varied considerably, for example, in France by 2003 and four years later in the UK, but by the end of the decade all affluent countries had introduced CF NBS.

6. Conclusions

This historical review focuses on the crucial stages in the development of a reliable neonatal screening test for the early detection of cystic fibrosis in the pre-symptomatic stages of this debilitating disease. Initiating this endeavour was the conviction of many paediatricians with expertise in the treatment of these patients, as the earlier a diagnosis was made, the better the clinical outcome. It seemed particularly fitting that 20 years of work undertaken to justify CF NBS should come to fruition at the beginning of a new millennium and that it should coincide with recent advances in CFTR molecular genetics. The better understanding of CFTR structural/functional relationships would undoubtedly pave the way for new and more effective treatments for CF children born in the 21st century, in addition to the benefits that NBS would provide. The generation of paediatricians and clinical biochemists who had pioneered this work internationally had reason to be satisfied with the outcome of their efforts. CF NBS had at last come of age. The inclusion of DNA in the post 1990 CF NBS protocols, was primarily to overcome a problem inherent in IRT–IRT, i.e., the need to retest about 1 in 250 infants at 2–3 weeks of age. Unanswered was the question—could IRT-DNA in the longer term present its own problems? Perhaps a review of CF NBS in the following decades will reveal the answer.

Funding: This research received no external funding.

Conflicts of Interest: The authors declare no conflict of interest.

References

1. Shwachman, H.; Kulczycki, L.L. Long-term study of 105 cystic fibrosis patients. *Am. J. Dis. Child.* **1958**, *96*, 6–15. [CrossRef] [PubMed]
2. Stephan, U.; Busch, E.W.; Kollberg, H.; Hellsing, K. Cystic fibrosis detection by means of a test-strip. *Pediatrics* **1975**, *55*, 35–38. [PubMed]
3. Evans, R.T.; Little, A.J.; Steel, A.E.; Littlewood, J.M. Satisfactory screening for cystic fibrosis with the BM meconium procedure. *J. Clin. Pathol.* **1981**, *34*, 911–913. [CrossRef] [PubMed]
4. Crossley, J.R.; Elliot, R.B.; Smith, P.A. Cystic Fibrosis screening in the newborn. *Lancet* **1979**, *i*, 1093–1095. [CrossRef]
5. Heeley, A.F.; Watson, D. Cystic Fibrosis—Its biochemical detection. *Clin. Chem.* **1983**, *29*, 2011–2018. [CrossRef]
6. Guthrie, R.; Susi, A. A simple phenylalanine method for detecting phenylketonuria in large populations of newborn infants. *Pediatrics* **1963**, *32*, 338–343.
7. Dussault, J.H.; Coulombe, P.; Laberge, J.; Guyda, H.; Khoury, K. Preliminary report on a mass screening program for neonatal hypothyroidism. *J. Pediatr.* **1975**, *86*, 670–674. [CrossRef]
8. Crossley, J.R.; Elliott, R.B.; Smith, P.A. Dried blood spot screening for cystic fibrosis in the newborn. *Lancet* **1979**, *i*, 472–474. [CrossRef]
9. King, D.N.; Heeley, A.F.; Walsh, M.P.; Kuzemko, J.A. Sensitive trypsin assay for dried blood specimens as a screening procedure for early detection of cystic fibrosis. *Lancet* **1979**, *ii*, 1217–1219. [CrossRef]
10. Carter, E.P.; Barrett, A.D.; Heeley, A.F.; Kuzemko, J.A. Improved sweat test method for the diagnosis of cystic fibrosis. *Arch. Dis. Child.* **1984**, *59*, 919–922. [CrossRef]
11. Heeley, A.F.; Heeley, M.E.; King, D.N.; Kuzemko, J.A.; Walsh, M.P. Screening for cystic fibrosis by dried blood spot trypsin assay. *Arch. Dis. Child.* **1982**, *57*, 18–21. [PubMed]
12. Travert, G.; Duhamel, J.F. Dépistage néonatal systématique de la mucoviscidose par dosage de la trypsine immunoréactive sanguine. Bilan de 80000 tests. *Arch. Fr. Pédiatr.* **1983**, *40*, 295–298. [PubMed]
13. Ryley, H.C.; Deam, S.M.; Williams, J.; Alfaham, M.; Weller, P.H.; Goodchild, M.C.; Carter, R.A.; Bradley, D.; Dodge, J.A. Neonatal screening for cystic fibrosis in Wales and the West Midlands: 1. Evaluation of immunoreactive trypsin. *J. Clin. Pathol.* **1988**, *41*, 726–729. [CrossRef] [PubMed]

14. Farrell, P.M.; Kosorok, M.R.; Rock, M.J.; Laxova, A.; Zeng, L.; Hoffman, G. Assessment of the benefits, risks and costs of cystic fibrosis screening in Wisconsin, USA. In Proceedings of the Neonatal Screening for Cystic Fibrosis, Caen, France, 10–11 September, 1998; Presses Universitaires de Caen, 1999; pp. 239–253.
15. Heeley, A.F.; Bangert, S.K. The neonatal detection of cystic fibrosis by measurement of immunoreactive trypsin in blood. *Ann. Clin. Biochem.* **1992**, *29*, 361–376. [CrossRef]
16. Wilcken, B. Newborn screening for cystic fibrosis; its evolution and a review of the current situation. *Screening* **1993**, *2*, 43–62. [CrossRef]
17. Heeley, M.E.; Travert, G.; Ferré, C.; Lemonnier, F. The International Quality Assurance Program for the assay of immunoreactive trypsin in dried blood spots. *Pediatr. Pulmonol.* **1991**, *11* (Suppl. 7), 72–75. [CrossRef]
18. Bowling, F.G.; Brown, A.R.D. Newborn screening for cystic fibrosis using an ELISA technique. *Clin. Chim. Acta* **1988**, *63*, 196–198.
19. Kerem, B.S.; Rommens, J.M.; Buchanan, J.A.; Markiewicz, D.; Cox, T.K.; Chakravarti, A.; Buchwald, M.; Tsui, L.C. Identification of the cystic fibrosis gene: Genetic analysis. *Science* **1989**, *245*, 1073–1080. [CrossRef]
20. Laroche, D.; Travert, G. The application of PCR amplification and the polymorphic marker KM19 to dried blood spots: Comparison with deletion F508 for the confirmation of the neonatal screening for cystic fibrosis. *Pediatr. Pulmonol.* **1991**, *11* (Suppl. 7), 19–22. [CrossRef]
21. Ranieri, E.; Ryall, R.G.; Robertson, E.E.; Pollard, A.C. A screening strategy for cystic fibrosis using immunoreactive trypsinogen and gene analysis. *Paediatric. Pulmonol.* **1991**, *Suppl 7*, 88. [CrossRef]
22. Pollitt, R.J.; Dalton, A.; Evans, S.; Boyne, J. *Three Stage Neonatal Screening (IRT-DNA-IRT) Neonatal Screening for Cystic Fibrosis*; Presses Universitaires de Caen: Caen, France, 1999; pp. 49–53.
23. Laroche, D.; Travert, G. Abnormal frequency of ΔF508 in neonatal transitory hypertrypsinaemia. *Lancet* **1991**, *337*, 55. [CrossRef]
24. Lecoq, I.; Brouard, J.; Laroche, D.; Férec, C.; Travert, G. Blood immunoreactive trypsinogen concentrations are genetically determined in healthy and cystic fibrosis newborns. *Acta Paediatr.* **1999**, *88*, 1–4. [CrossRef]
25. Kuzemko, J.A. Clinical Implications of screening for cystic fibrosis in the newborn. *Insights into Paediatr.* **1987**, *1*, 1–87, Gardiner-Caldwell, Macclesfield, UK.
26. *Neonatal Screening for Cystic Fibrosis*; Presses Universitaires de Caen: Caen, France, 1999; ISBN 2-84133-075-3.
27. Available online: http://cfmedicine.com/history (accessed on 30 January 2020).

© 2020 by the authors. Licensee MDPI, Basel, Switzerland. This article is an open access article distributed under the terms and conditions of the Creative Commons Attribution (CC BY) license (http://creativecommons.org/licenses/by/4.0/).

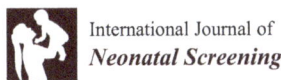

International Journal of
Neonatal Screening

Review

The Changing Face of Cystic Fibrosis and Its Implications for Screening

Lutz Naehrlich

Department of Pediatrics, Justus-Liebig-University Giessen, D-35392 Giessen, Germany; lutz.naehrlich@paediat.med.uni-giessen.de; Tel.: +49-641-9857621

Received: 22 May 2020; Accepted: 30 June 2020; Published: 3 July 2020

Abstract: Early diagnosis, multidisciplinary care, and optimized and preventive treatments have changed the face of cystic fibrosis. Life expectancy has been expanded in the last decades. Formerly a pediatric disease, cystic fibrosis has reached adulthood. Mutation-specific treatments will expand treatment options and give hope for further improvement of quality of life and life expectancy. Newborn screening for CF fits perfectly into these care structures and offers the possibility of preventive treatment even before symptoms occur. Especially in countries without screening, newborn screening will fulfill that promise only with increased awareness and new care structures.

Keywords: cystic fibrosis; newborn screening; diagnosis; therapy; prognosis

1. Introduction

Cystic fibrosis (CF) is a life-shortening multisystem disease with an autosomal recessive inheritance pattern that affects nearly 100,000, mainly Caucasian, people worldwide. The disease is caused by dysfunction of the exocrine gland chloride channel protein, the cystic fibrosis transmembrane conductance regulator (*CFTR*). CF mainly involves the pancreas and the lungs, but also the upper airways, liver, intestine, skin, and reproductive organs. Improved diagnosis, a multidisciplinary team approach, and symptomatic treatment have improved the health and survival prospects of persons with CF. Early diagnosis by newborn screening (NBS) [1] and prophylactic treatment are critical components for overall success. The approval of causally directed, mutation-specific treatments creates hope for reduced morbidity and increased life expectancy in the near future. The face of CF has changed over the last decades. This has implications for CF NBS, especially in countries in which it is not yet established.

2. Changing Face of Cystic Fibrosis

2.1. Diagnosis

Since the first description of CF [2,3] in the 1930s, clinical and pathophysiological knowledge and diagnostic and therapeutic possibilities have changed and influenced each other. In the beginning, CF was diagnosed based on clinical symptoms, such as meconium ileus, exocrine pancreatic insufficiency, chronic pneumonia, or post-mortem findings of cystic fibrosis of the pancreas and the lung [2]. During a heat wave in New York in 1948, disturbances of electrolytes were detected in CF patients [4]. The increased sweat chloride concentration was described in 1953 as a characteristic finding in CF, [5] and since then has been used as a diagnostic tool. In 1959, Gibson and Cooke published a method for sweat induction by pilocarpine iontophoresis on a small body surface area [6], and it remains the diagnostic gold standard for CF even today. Measuring conductivity by Nanoduct® can facilitate the diagnosis of screening-positive newborns, but is less specific than the sweat chloride measurement [7] and not recommended as a diagnostic measurement [8].

A close observation of families with CF led to its description as an autosomal recessive genetic disorder in 1946 [9]. In 1989, the cystic fibrosis gene on the long arm of chromosome 7 was identified [10], paving the way for genetic diagnosis. To date, more than 2000 *CFTR* mutations have been described (http://www.genet.sickkids.on.ca) [11]. Functional and clinical analyses have led to the characterization of 432 variants, including 352 disease–causing variants (https://www.cftr2.org) [12] and the concept of functional mutation classes [13]. Worldwide, F508del is the major CF variant, but the prevalence varies between ethnic groups (for example, 70% in Germany and 25% in Turkey) [14]. Despite extensive *CFTR* sequencing, around 1% of *CFTR* variants have not been identified. To confirm the diagnosis in these cases, in vivo functional *CFTR* testing, such as nasal potential difference measurement and intestinal current measurement were implemented [8].

Due to the consistent clinical characterization of CF patients, the first pancreatic-sufficient CF patients were reported in the 1950s [15]. This group of patients, characterized by *CFTR* mutations with residual *CFTR* function, accounts for 10–15% of all CF patients [16]. They can present with similar severity of lung disease, but as a group have a better prognosis than others. In 1975, the first pancreatic-insufficient CF patient with a normal sweat chloride test was reported [17]. A normal sweat chloride test was reported in 3.5% of all patients in the US in 2015 [18], these patients were diagnosed based on two CF-causing mutations or pathologic CFTR functional tests. In the 1990s, the first CF diagnoses in adolescents and adults were reported [19]. The patients are mainly pancreatic sufficient but infertile due to an obstructive azoospermia and suffer from respiratory symptoms [19]. In Germany, 5% of all CF-patients are diagnosed at age 18 years or older [20]. The expanding knowledge of patients with a clinical entity associated with CFTR-dysfunction that does not fulfill the diagnostic criteria for CF widened the spectrum and led to the description of *CFTR*-related disorders [21]. International guidelines [8] have been updated regularly and reflect the expanding knowledge of the spectrum of *CFTR* dysfunction and the widely varying clinical presentation of CF.

2.2. Care

CF care today is seen as multidisciplinary, to fit the medical, psychosocial, physiotherapeutic, and nutritional needs of CF patients, prevent chronic infection and malnutrition, minimize deterioration, maintain independence, optimize quality of life, and maximize life expectancy [22].

Until the 1950s, many pediatricians took care of CF-patients, and only a few doctors, those dedicated to CF, treated more than a handful of patients. Broader experience with the spectrum of the disease and rare complications, the ability to analyze treatment options and outcome in a more systematic way, and long-term follow-up are the major advantages of CF-center care and also drive clinical research and progress. In 1958, Shwachmann and Kulczycki published their results from a large cohort of 105 patients, marking the beginning of center-based care worldwide [23]. The Cystic Fibrosis Foundation in the USA established an accredited care network in 1961 by creating centers devoted to treating CF. The number of Foundation-accredited care centers in the USA grew to more than 100 by 1978 and there are currently 130 (https://www.cff.org/About-Us/About-the-Cystic-Fibrosis-Foundation/Our-History/). In 1963, the CFF Foundation published the first guidelines for the diagnosis and treatment of CF. These achievements inspired colleagues and parents to establish a national CF foundation and CF care centers across the world and to deliver structured care, including annual checkups and regular outpatient visits [24]. The integration of clinical research reflected by the establishment of clinical trial networks in the USA, Canada, and Europe have sped up the development of clinical trials [25]. This combination of clinical research and best care practices has been cited as a model of effective and efficient healthcare delivery for other chronic diseases. A transition from pediatric to adult care began in the 1960s with the increasing number of adults with CF, but it is still a challenge globally.

2.3. Therapy

The paradigm for comprehensive and preventive treatment programs for CF was introduced by Matthews, who first suggested and funded a program in 1957 in Cleveland [26]. Accurate early diagnosis and treatment from diagnosis had a dramatic impact on survival and morbidity at this time. This paradigm has been adopted globally and is the basis of our Standards of Care today [24]. The evolution of the diagnostic and therapeutic Standards of Care for CF was based on clinical experience and controlled studies. Until the 1990s, almost all therapeutic strategies for CF were based on center experiences and comparisons with historical controls. Since then, drug development has been based mainly on randomized placebo-controlled studies. Neither strategy answers all relevant clinical questions, and both leave room for interpretation and individual treatment regimens.

The symptomatic treatment of pancreatic insufficiency, which affects 85–90% of all CF patients, started in the 1930s (in the absence of pancreatic enzyme replacement) as a low-fat, high-protein diet. Pancreatic enzyme replacement was established in the 1940s, but required high doses due to the enzymes' lack of resistance to gastric acid. After gastric-acid resistant pancreatic enzyme therapy was established in the 1980s based on a historical comparison of center data, dietary recommendations changed from a low-fat diet to a high-fat, high-calorie diet. Instead of a standard dosage regimen, individual dosage adjustment of pancreatic enzymes and fat-soluble vitamins and nutritional advice from a specialized dietician are critical to overcoming malnutrition and achieving sufficient blood vitamin levels [27].

Symptomatic mucolytic therapy today is mainly based on inhalation of DNase [28], hypertonic saline, [29] or mannitol [30] in combination with physiotherapy. High quality studies comparing the mucolytic drugs are still lacking, and the individual experiences of patients and caregivers explain the high variability of their use globally. Mucolytic therapy was shown to reduce pulmonary exacerbation frequency and to improve and stabilize lung function. Physiotherapy is an important daily prophylactic and therapeutic component of care, and is based on personalized experience and different approaches [24].

Chronic bacterial pneumonia has been a continuous challenge for CF care since the first description of CF. *Staphylococcus aureus* and *Pseudomonas aeruginosa* (PA) are the most important bugs [18]. The concept of early detection and eradication of *P. aeruginosa* was established in the 1990s in order to postpone chronic infection [31], which is defined by more than 50% of the preceding 12 months being PA culture positive [32]. Methicillin resistant *Staphylococcus aureus* and nontuberculous mycobacteria are emerging pathogens in CF [18]. Aggressive antibiotic treatment of pulmonary exacerbations is the backbone of pulmonary treatment. Lower treatment thresholds, higher dosages, and longer treatment durations compared with those typical for non-CF patients are mainly based on clinical experience. Chronic suppression therapy by inhalation of antibiotics was first described in the 1980s [33]. A placebo-controlled trial in the 1990s confirmed the concept [34]. Infection control at home and in the hospital are critical components of avoidance of both cross-infection and infection with multi-resistant bugs. These concepts have been defined in the last 10 years and contribute to the control of chronic bacterial infection in CF.

The active surveillance of CF-related complications, such as liver disease, diabetes mellitus, bone disease, and their active treatments have become important components of annual checkups and therapeutic concepts [24]. Lung transplantation has a major impact on survival. In France and Belgium, 10–13% of all CF patients have undergone lung transplantation, compared to less than 2% in most eastern European countries [16].

In the last decade, causally directed, mutation-specific treatments have been evolving. In contrast to gene therapy, [35] orally administered small molecules with systemic effects have been shown to increase CFTR function (reducing sweat chloride), lung function, body weight, and quality of life significantly. These effects depend highly on the particular drugs, which are divided into correctors and modulators, and the mutation classes. The proof of concept has been shown with Ivacaftor for patients with at least one gating mutation (3% of all CF patients in Europe) [36–38]. This treatment is licensed in the European Union (EU) for use from the age of 6 months. Ivacaftor treatment in children aged 12 to 24 months with a gating mutation support the potential of Ivacaftor to protect against progressive exocrine pancreatic dysfunction [38]. In utero treatment provided partial protection from pathologies in pancreas, intestine, and male reproductive tract in a ferret model [39]. A combination of Elexacaftor/Tezacaftor/Ivacaftor has shown comparable data in patients with at least one F508del mutation (90% of all patients in Europe) [40,41]. This drug was licensed in the USA in 2019 for patients older than 12 years of age, and the decision of the European Medical Agency is expected in 2020. Another combination, of Lumacaftor/Ivacaftor, is licensed in the EU for F508del homozygous patients (45% of all patients in Europe) for use from the age of 2 years [42], but its effect is limited compared with Elexacaftor/Tezacaftor/Ivacaftor. All these trial developments are the result of close cooperation between clinical trial networks, CF centers, and industry, and the drugs have been tested as an add-on to the standard symptomatic therapy. These developments offer great hope for parents of newborns with CF by improving quality of life and life expectancy in the near future.

2.4. Prognosis

CF was seen as a pediatric disease for many decades, affecting only a few adult patients. This has changed dramatically since the 1990s. With reduced pediatric morbidity and mortality, more pediatric patients are surviving to adulthood [43]. For example, the rate of malnutrition declined from 26% to 17% in children and adolescents and from 26% to 14% in adults in Germany from 2009 to 2018 [20,44]. The rate of chronic *Pseudomonas* infection in 16–19-year-old patients dropped from 43.9% in 2009 to 25.5% in 2018 in the UK [45]. Nearly 40% of all adults 18–29 years of age had normal lung function (FEV1%pred) of more than 80% in 2017, compared with 30% in 2008/2009 in Europe [16,46].

During the last decades, great improvements in survival were achieved. In 1980, 31.1 % of the US CF population was over the age of 18 years, compared with 54.6% in 2018. In Belgium, Denmark, Netherland, Norway, and Sweden, adults were reported to make up 60–65% of all CF patients in 2017 [16]. This comes with dramatic improvements in increasing the age of death, survival of birth cohorts, and median survival age over time [43]. For the period 2012–2016, the median age of survival was estimated to be 53.3 (95% CI: unknown) in Canada, 47.5 years (95% CI: 44.8–49.7) in Germany, 47.0 years (95% CI: 44.7–48.2) in the UK, and 42.7 years (95% CI: 41.7–43.9) in the USA [47].

These improvements have far-reaching implications in terms of care structures and resources. To fulfill the increasingly promising prognosis, access to care including dedicated multidisciplinary CF teams and a broad range of medicines is critical. Socioeconomic status (SES) is a major confounder and must be taken into account. Studies in the USA have found that medical insurance status [48] and median household income [49] are both independently associated with significant differences in survival, even within a country with a high mean gross net income. Comparing the highest SES countries with the lowest SES countries in Europe showed a significant decrease in the hazard of mortality [50].

3. Implications for Newborn Screening

Despite the continuously improving quality of life and life expectancy of patients over the last decades and promising therapeutic developments, CF is still a chronic, life-limiting disease. Early diagnosis and multidisciplinary treatment according to current standards of care are critical in avoiding early severe complications. The following are some key implications of screening that must be discussed.

The awareness of cystic fibrosis in general, but especially of the improving prognosis and treatment options, is critical for the success of NBS. The common problems of late diagnosis and underdiagnosis in some countries reflect the low awareness of CF among caregivers, parents, and health authorities. The promising prognosis has to be emphasized. Patient representatives and organizations could help to support this important public health topic by personalizing experiences and helping to create a supportive environment for families after diagnosis. CF caregivers are responsible for advocacy for CF, especially among healthcare professionals, and for providing obstetricians, surgeons, pediatricians, and general practitioners with updated information about CF in general, the spectrum of disease presentation, diagnostic and therapeutic options, and improving overall prognosis. Patient registries are important tools for collecting, reporting, and comparing international and national epidemiologic data. CF caregivers and patient organizations should jointly stand up to raise awareness (and resources) amongst health authorities, provide information about medical needs, and discuss and propose care structures for each country.

CF core diagnostic and care facilities with established multidisciplinary teams must be established and promoted in each country. Pediatric facilities should be integrated within a NBS tracking system and take an active role in providing information to local caregivers, patients, and health authorities. The confirmation of the diagnosis should be performed at the earliest stage in specialized CF centers. The results have to be discussed by a CF experienced doctor on the day the diagnosis is confirmed. Critical components of the service are a high-quality sweat chloride test to minimize the rate of sweat tests with insufficient volume and give reliable results on the day of the confirmation visit, a multidisciplinary team to counsel the parents and establish the treatment plan immediately, and strict infection control to minimize the risk of *P. aeruginosa* acquisition. Without this essential infrastructure, even the best NBS program cannot succeed [51].

High specificity of the newborn screening program reduces the recall rate, the parents' burden and stress, and the burden of CF centers. Due to the low number of CF centers in some countries, the travel distance and burden for families should not be underestimated. The genetic component of each individual NBS program is critical to achieving the goal. The selection of mutations for screening has to be adapted to the genetic and ethnic spectrum of each country/region and could be based on registry data or epidemiologic studies. The detection of mutations with varying consequences through newborn screening should be avoided as it will complicate interpretation and overextend caregivers and patients. An expanded mutation panel or genotyping should not be "abused" to substitute for robust confirmation of diagnosis. Unfortunately, commercial panel testing does not fit this need. Measuring pancreatitis associated protein in addition to immunoreactive trypsinogen might be an additional 2nd tier to reduce the use of genetic analyses [52]. Learning from international experience is the best way to build up individual NBS programs for each country. Even the best CF screening program will not detect all patients at birth, and awareness of the possibility of later diagnosis is needed anyway.

Changes in diagnostic and therapeutic dogmas are driven fundamentally by NBS. Unlike symptomatic patients who are diagnosed by confirmation of *CFTR* dysfunction, asymptomatic patients are diagnosed based on proven *CFTR* dysfunction. In contrast to symptomatic treatment, which is often well received and accepted by parents, the diagnosis and prophylactic treatment of asymptomatic children is often mistrusted and seen as a greater burden by parents. The developing mutation-specific treatments offer great hope for parents of newborns with CF. Only if healthcare providers (including primary care providers) and parents are convinced and have hope that early diagnosis and treatment offers a benefit for the patient, such as avoiding or postponing malnutrition or pulmonary and other complications, will NBS fulfill its promise.

4. Conclusions

NBS for CF should be seen as a game changer in CF care, not reduced to simply a diagnostic procedure. Its final success depends on the general awareness of the disease, the integration of NBS within well-established CF care structures, and the engagement and interaction of obstetricians, primary caregivers, pediatricians, CF centers, and health authorities.

Funding: This research received no external funding.

Conflicts of Interest: The author declares no conflict of interest.

References

1. Castellani, C.; Massie, J.; Sontag, M.; Southern, K.W. Newborn screening for cystic fibrosis. *Lancet Respir. Med.* **2016**, *4*, 653–661. [CrossRef]
2. Andersen, D.H. Cystic fibrosis of the pancreas and its relation to celiac disease: A clinical and pathological study. *Am. J. Dis. Child.* **1938**, *56*, 344–399. [CrossRef]
3. Fanconi, G.; Uehlinger, E.; Knauer, C. Das Coeliakie-syndrom bei angeborener zystischer Pankreasfibromatose und Bronchiektasien. *Wien. Med. Wchnschr* **1936**, *86*, 753–756.
4. Kessler, W.R.; Andersen, D.H. Heat prostration in fibrocystic disease of the pancreas and other conditions. *Pediatrics* **1951**, *8*, 648–656.
5. Di Sant'Agnese, P.A.; Darling, R.C.; Perera, G.A.; Shea, E. Abnormal electrolyte composition of sweat in cystic fibrosis of the pancreas; clinical significance and relationship to the disease. *Pediatrics* **1953**, *12*, 549–563.
6. Gibson, L.E.; Cooke, R.E. A test for concentration of electrolytes in sweat in cystic fibrosis of the pancreas utilizing pilocarpine by iontophoresis. *Pediatrics* **1959**, *23*, 545–549. [PubMed]
7. Rueegg, C.S.; Kuehni, C.E.; Gallati, S.; Jurca, M.; Jung, A.; Casaulta, C.; Barben, J. Comparison of two sweat test systems for the diagnosis of cystic fibrosis in newborns. *Pediatr. Pulmonol.* **2019**, *54*, 264–272. [CrossRef] [PubMed]
8. Farrell, P.M.; White, T.B.; Howenstine, M.S.; Munck, A.; Parad, R.B.; Rosenfeld, M.; Sommerburg, O.; Accurso, F.J.; Davies, J.C.; Rock, M.J.; et al. Diagnosis of Cystic Fibrosis in Screened Populations. *J. Pediatr.* **2017**, *181*, S33–S44.e2. [CrossRef] [PubMed]
9. Andersen, D.H.; Hodges, R.G. Celiac syndrome; genetics of cystic fibrosis of the pancreas, with a consideration of etiology. *Am. J. Dis. Child.* **1946**, *72*, 62–80. [CrossRef] [PubMed]
10. Kerem, B.; Rommens, J.M.; Buchanan, J.A.; Markiewicz, D.; Cox, T.K.; Chakravarti, A.; Buchwald, M.; Tsui, L.C. Identification of the cystic fibrosis gene: Genetic analysis. *Science* **1989**, *245*, 1073–1080. [CrossRef]
11. Cystic Fibrosis Mutation Database (CFTR1). Available online: http://www.genet.sickkids.on.ca (accessed on 17 May 2020).
12. Sosnay, P.R.; Siklosi, K.R.; Van Goor, F.; Kaniecki, K.; Yu, H.; Sharma, N.; Ramalho, A.S.; Amaral, M.D.; Dorfman, R.; Zielenski, J.; et al. Defining the disease liability of variants in the cystic fibrosis transmembrane conductance regulator gene. *Nat. Genet.* **2013**, *45*, 1160–1167. [CrossRef] [PubMed]
13. Boyle, M.P.; De Boeck, K. A new era in the treatment of cystic fibrosis: Correction of the underlying CFTR defect. *Lancet Respir. Med.* **2013**, *1*, 158–163. [CrossRef]
14. World Health Organization. The Molecular Genetic Epidemiology of Cystic Fibrosis. Available online: http://www.who.int/genomics/publications/reports/en/index.html (accessed on 29 June 2020).
15. Dooley, R.R.; Guilmette, F.; Leubner, H.; Patterson, P.R.; Shwachman, H.; Weil, C. Cystic fibrosis of the pancreas with varying degrees of pancreatic insufficiency. *AMA J. Dis. Child.* **1956**, *92*, 347–368. [PubMed]
16. Zolin, A.; Orenti, A.; Naehrlich, L.; van Rens, J.; Fox, A.; Krasnyk, M.; Jung, A.; Mei-Zahav, M.; Cosgriff, R.; Storms, V.; et al. *ECFSPR Annual Report 2017*; European Cystic Fibrosis Society: Karup, Denmark, 2019.
17. Sarsfield, J.K.; Davies, J.M. Negative sweat tests and cystic fibrosis. *Arch. Dis. Child.* **1975**, *50*, 463–466. [CrossRef] [PubMed]
18. Cystic Fibrosis Foundation. *Cystic Fibrosis Foundation Patient Registry—2015 Annual Data Report*; Cystic Fibrosis Foundation: Bethesda, MD, USA, 2016.
19. Gan, K.H.; Geus, W.P.; Bakker, W.; Lamers, C.B.; Heijerman, H.G. Genetic and clinical features of patients with cystic fibrosis diagnosed after the age of 16 years. *Thorax* **1995**, *50*, 1301–1304. [CrossRef]
20. Nährlich, L.; Burkhart, M.; Wosniok, J. *German Cystic Fibrosis registry—Annual Report 2018*; Mukoviszidose Institut GmbH: Bonn, Germany, 2019.
21. Bombieri, C.; Claustres, M.; De Boeck, K.; Derichs, N.; Dodge, J.; Girodon, E.; Sermet, I.; Schwarz, M.; Tzetis, M.; Wilschanski, M.; et al. Recommendations for the classification of diseases as CFTR-related disorders. *J. Cyst. Fibros.* **2011**, *10*, S86–S102. [CrossRef]
22. Smyth, A.R.; Bell, S.C.; Bojcin, S.; Bryon, M.; Duff, A.; Flume, P.; Kashirskaya, N.; Munck, A.; Ratjen, F.; Schwarzenberg, S.J.; et al. European Cystic Fibrosis Society Standards of Care: Best Practice guidelines. *J. Cyst. Fibros.* **2014**, *13*, S23–S42. [CrossRef]
23. Shwachman, H.; Kulczycki, L.L. Long-term study of one hundred five patients with cystic fibrosis; studies made over a five- to fourteen-year period. *AMA J. Dis. Child.* **1958**, *96*, 6–15. [CrossRef]

24. Castellani, C.; Duff, A.J.A.; Bell, S.C.; Heijerman, H.G.M.; Munck, A.; Ratjen, F.; Sermet-Gaudelus, I.; Southern, K.W.; Barben, J.; Flume, P.A.; et al. ECFS best practice guidelines: The 2018 revision. *J. Cyst. Fibros.* **2018**, *17*, 153–178. [CrossRef]
25. De Boeck, K.; Bulteel, V.; Fajac, I. Disease-specific clinical trials networks: The example of cystic fibrosis. *Eur. J. Pediatr.* **2016**, *175*, 817–824. [CrossRef]
26. Doershuk, C.F.; Matthews, L.W.; Tucker, A.S.; Nudleman, H.; Eddy, G.; Wise, M.; Spector, S. A 5year clinical evaluation of a therapeutic program for patients with cystic fibrosis. *J. Pediatr.* **1964**, *65*, 677–693. [CrossRef]
27. Turck, D.; Braegger, C.P.; Colombo, C.; Declercq, D.; Morton, A.; Pancheva, R.; Robberecht, E.; Stern, M.; Strandvik, B.; Wolfe, S.; et al. ESPEN-ESPGHAN-ECFS guidelines on nutrition care for infants, children, and adults with cystic fibrosis. *Clin. Nutr.* **2016**, *35*, 557–577. [CrossRef] [PubMed]
28. Yang, C.; Chilvers, M.; Montgomery, M.; Nolan, S.J. Dornase alfa for cystic fibrosis. *Cochrane Database Syst. Rev.* **2016**, *4*, Cd001127. [CrossRef]
29. Wark, P.; McDonald, V.M. Nebulised hypertonic saline for cystic fibrosis. *Cochrane Database Syst. Rev.* **2009**, *15*, Cd001506. [CrossRef] [PubMed]
30. Nolan, S.J.; Thornton, J.; Murray, C.S.; Dwyer, T. Inhaled mannitol for cystic fibrosis. *Cochrane Database Syst. Rev.* **2015**, *10*, Cd008649. [CrossRef]
31. Valerius, N.H.; Koch, C.; Hoiby, N. Prevention of chronic Pseudomonas aeruginosa colonisation in cystic fibrosis by early treatment. *Lancet* **1991**, *338*, 725–726. [CrossRef]
32. Lee, T.W.; Brownlee, K.G.; Conway, S.P.; Denton, M.; Littlewood, J.M. Evaluation of a new definition for chronic Pseudomonas aeruginosa infection in cystic fibrosis patients. *J. Cyst. Fibros.* **2003**, *2*, 29–34. [CrossRef]
33. Jensen, T.; Pedersen, S.S.; Garne, S.; Heilmann, C.; Hoiby, N.; Koch, C. Colistin inhalation therapy in cystic fibrosis patients with chronic Pseudomonas aeruginosa lung infection. *J. Antimicrob. Chemother.* **1987**, *19*, 831–838. [CrossRef]
34. Ramsey, B.W.; Pepe, M.S.; Quan, J.M.; Otto, K.L.; Montgomery, A.B.; Williams-Warren, J.; Vasiljev, K.M.; Borowitz, D.; Bowman, C.M.; Marshall, B.C.; et al. Intermittent administration of inhaled tobramycin in patients with cystic fibrosis. Cystic Fibrosis Inhaled Tobramycin Study Group. *N. Engl. J. Med.* **1999**, *340*, 23–30. [CrossRef]
35. Alton, E.; Armstrong, D.K.; Ashby, D.; Bayfield, K.J.; Bilton, D.; Bloomfield, E.V.; Boyd, A.C.; Brand, J.; Buchan, R.; Calcedo, R.; et al. Repeated nebulisation of non-viral CFTR gene therapy in patients with cystic fibrosis: A randomised, double-blind, placebo-controlled, phase 2b trial. *Lancet Respir. Med.* **2015**, *3*, 684–691. [CrossRef]
36. Ramsey, B.W.; Davies, J.; McElvaney, N.G.; Tullis, E.; Bell, S.C.; Drevinek, P.; Griese, M.; McKone, E.F.; Wainwright, C.E.; Konstan, M.W.; et al. A CFTR potentiator in patients with cystic fibrosis and the G551D mutation. *N. Engl. J. Med.* **2011**, *365*, 1663–1672. [CrossRef] [PubMed]
37. Davies, J.C.; Wainwright, C.E.; Canny, G.J.; Chilvers, M.A.; Howenstine, M.S.; Munck, A.; Mainz, J.G.; Rodriguez, S.; Li, H.; Yen, K.; et al. Efficacy and safety of ivacaftor in patients aged 6 to 11 years with cystic fibrosis with a G551D mutation. *Am. J. Respir. Crit. Care Med.* **2013**, *187*, 1219–1225. [CrossRef] [PubMed]
38. Rosenfeld, M.; Wainwright, C.E.; Higgins, M.; Wang, L.T.; McKee, C.; Campbell, D.; Tian, S.; Schneider, J.; Cunningham, S.; Davies, J.C. Ivacaftor treatment of cystic fibrosis in children aged 12 to <24 months and with a CFTR gating mutation (ARRIVAL): A phase 3 single-arm study. *Lancet Respir. Med.* **2018**, *6*, 545–553. [CrossRef]
39. Sun, X.; Yi, Y.; Yan, Z.; Rosen, B.H.; Liang, B.; Winter, M.C.; Evans, T.I.A.; Rotti, P.G.; Yang, Y.; Gray, J.S.; et al. In utero and postnatal VX-770 administration rescues multiorgan disease in a ferret model of cystic fibrosis. *Sci. Transl. Med.* **2019**, *11*, eaau7531. [CrossRef] [PubMed]
40. Heijerman, H.G.M.; McKone, E.F.; Downey, D.G.; Van Braeckel, E.; Rowe, S.M.; Tullis, E.; Mall, M.A.; Welter, J.J.; Ramsey, B.W.; McKee, C.M.; et al. Efficacy and safety of the elexacaftor plus tezacaftor plus ivacaftor combination regimen in people with cystic fibrosis homozygous for the F508del mutation: A double-blind, randomised, phase 3 trial. *Lancet* **2019**, *394*, 1940–1948. [CrossRef]
41. Middleton, P.G.; Mall, M.A.; Drevinek, P.; Lands, L.C.; McKone, E.F.; Polineni, D.; Ramsey, B.W.; Taylor-Cousar, J.L.; Tullis, E.; Vermeulen, F.; et al. Elexacaftor-Tezacaftor-Ivacaftor for Cystic Fibrosis with a Single Phe508del Allele. *N. Engl. J. Med.* **2019**, *381*, 1809–1819. [CrossRef]

42. Ratjen, F.; Hug, C.; Marigowda, G.; Tian, S.; Huang, X.; Stanojevic, S.; Milla, C.E.; Robinson, P.D.; Waltz, D.; Davies, J.C. Efficacy and safety of lumacaftor and ivacaftor in patients aged 6-11 years with cystic fibrosis homozygous for F508del-CFTR: A randomised, placebo-controlled phase 3 trial. *Lancet Respir. Med.* **2017**, *5*, 557–567. [CrossRef]
43. Stephenson, A.L.; Stanojevic, S.; Sykes, J.; Burgel, P.R. The changing epidemiology and demography of cystic fibrosis. *Presse Med.* **2017**, *46*, e87–e95. [CrossRef]
44. Stern, M.; Sens, B.; Wiedemann, B.; Busse, O.; Damm, G.; Wenzlaff, P. *Qualitätssicherung Mukoviszidose—Überblick über den Gesundheitszustand der Patienten in Deutschland 2009*; Hippocampus-Verlag: Bad Honnef, Germany, 2010.
45. UK Cystic Fibrosis Registry. *Annual Data Report 2018.*; Cystic Fibrosis Trust: London, UK, 2019.
46. Vivani, L.; Zolin, A.; Olesen, H. *ECFSPR Annual Report 2008–2009*; European Cystic Fibrosis Society: Karup, Denmark, 2012.
47. Naehrlich, L. Survival analyis of the German Cystic Fibrosis Registry. *J. Cyst. Fibros.* **2019**, *18*, S75. [CrossRef]
48. Schechter, M.S.; Shelton, B.J.; Margolis, P.A.; Fitzsimmons, S.C. The association of socioeconomic status with outcomes in cystic fibrosis patients in the United States. *Am. J. Respir. Crit. Care Med.* **2001**, *163*, 1331–1337. [CrossRef]
49. O'Connor, G.T.; Quinton, H.B.; Kneeland, T.; Kahn, R.; Lever, T.; Maddock, J.; Robichaud, P.; Detzer, M.; Swartz, D.R. Median household income and mortality rate in cystic fibrosis. *Pediatrics* **2003**, *111*, e333–e339. [CrossRef] [PubMed]
50. McKone, E.; Ariti, C.; Jackson, A.; Zolin, A.; Carr, S.; VanRens, J.; Colomb, V.; Lemonnier, L.; Keogh, R.; Naehrlich, L. Cystic fibrosis survival and socioeconomic status across Europe. *J. Cyst. Fibros.* **2017**, *16*, S20. [CrossRef]
51. Barreda, C.B.; Farrell, P.M.; Laxova, A.; Eickhoff, J.C.; Braun, A.T.; Coller, R.J.; Rock, M.J. Newborn screening alone insufficient to improve pulmonary outcomes for cystic fibrosis. *J. Cyst. Fibros.* **2020**. [CrossRef] [PubMed]
52. Sommerburg, O.; Krulisova, V.; Hammermann, J.; Lindner, M.; Stahl, M.; Muckenthaler, M.; Kohlmueller, D.; Happich, M.; Kulozik, A.E.; Votava, F.; et al. Comparison of different IRT-PAP protocols to screen newborns for cystic fibrosis in three central European populations. *J. Cyst. Fibros.* **2014**, *13*, 15–23. [CrossRef]

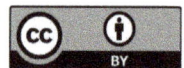

© 2020 by the author. Licensee MDPI, Basel, Switzerland. This article is an open access article distributed under the terms and conditions of the Creative Commons Attribution (CC BY) license (http://creativecommons.org/licenses/by/4.0/).

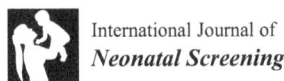
International Journal of
Neonatal Screening

Review

It All Depends What You Count—The Importance of Definitions in Evaluation of CF Screening Performance

Natasha Heather [1,2,*] and Dianne Webster [1,2]

1. National Newborn Metabolic Screening programme, LabPlus, Auckland City Hospital, Auckland 1148, New Zealand; diannew@adhb.govt.nz
2. Liggins Institute, University of Auckland, Auckland 1023, New Zealand
* Correspondence: NHeather@adhb.govt.nz

Received: 15 May 2020; Accepted: 8 June 2020; Published: 10 June 2020

Abstract: Screening metrics are essential to both quality assessment and improvement, but are highly dependent on the way positive tests and cases are counted. In cystic fibrosis (CF) screening, key factors include how mild cases of late-presenting CF and CF screen positive, inconclusive diagnosis (CFSPID) are counted, whether those at prior increased risk of CF are excluded from the screened population, and which aspects of the screening pathway are considered. This paper draws on the New Zealand experience of almost forty years of newborn screening for CF. We demonstrate how different definitions impact the calculation of screening sensitivity. We suggest that, to enable meaningful comparison, CF screening reports should clarify what steps in the screening pathway are included in the assessment, as well as the algorithm used and screening target.

Keywords: newborn screen; target disorder; missed case; sensitivity; cystic fibrosis; CFSPID; immunoreactive trypsin; meconium ileus

---

1. Introduction

Most newborn screening programmes want to know how they are performing. Local metrics, such as transit times for samples or the efficiency of short-term followup of unsuitable samples, are influenced by local conditions and can usefully be compared from time to time within a programme. Global metrics such as those used in public health (e.g., screening sensitivity, specificity, and positive predictive value) are widely used to compare performance between programmes. However, the comparison may not be based on equivalent counting of positive tests and detected and missed cases. This article explores the different definitions used in cystic fibrosis (CF) screening and the effects on screening metrics.

2. Factors to Consider

2.1. Target Disorder

When newborn screening started in the 1960s the understanding of disease was simpler—a baby either had PKU or not. As time went by it was recognized that a milder form existed and the baby had PKU or hyperphenylalaninemia. Then it became clear the borders between these conditions were not sharp, and considerable effort (phenylalanine loads) went into deciding whether a baby with a raised phenylalanine level had hyperphenylalaninemia type one to five (from benign to severe). Finally, the spectrum of disease was recognized, and now it is considered that each person with raised blood phenylalanine has their own disease determined not only by variants in the phenylalanine hydroxylase gene but also by other protein-metabolizing and amino acid-transporting systems.

Similarly, at the time that screening for CF started in the late 1970s [1] it was considered to be a uniformly serious childhood condition. However, since the discovery of the cystic fibrosis transmembrane regulator (CFTR) [2], the CF phenotype has been broadened to include mild and late-presenting disease, such as otherwise healthy males presenting with infertility and older adults with mild respiratory symptoms but found to carry two "pathogenic" CFTR variants [3]. Many CF screening programmes have only been in place for a few years. The recognition of a broadened CF phenotype has created problems in defining the outcome as well as the target of screening.

The biological level at which screening and confirmatory investigations are performed (genetic and/or functional assessment) impacts the number and severity of cases that will be detected [4]. The 2017 CF Foundation consensus guidelines reinforce the importance of a sweat test in establishing a diagnosis of CF [5]. The NewSTEPS case definition acknowledges that a sweat test is the gold standard, but accepts that a diagnosis could also be established by genotyping [6]. Furthermore, most screening programmes would say that a detected case is an infant with a positive newborn screen who went on to be diagnosed with CF. However, some infants have ambiguous genotypes (e.g., one pathogenic variant and another variant of unknown significance) and/or biochemical phenotypes (low but still abnormal sweat chlorides, such as 30–59 mmol/L) and may or may not develop classical CF symptoms later. These infants are now described as CF screen positive, inconclusive diagnosis (CFSPID) [7,8].

This raises the question—what is a diagnosis? When an infant presents with meconium ileus or failure to thrive, the diagnosis is CF. When an infant has a positive screen, confirmatory tests (sweat and pancreatic function) and possibly previously unidentified clinical features can also lead to the early diagnosis of CF. However, infants with CFSPID are apparently healthy, asymptomatic infants who are essentially diagnosed based on their newborn screen, as further tests have been inconclusive. CFSPID sounds like a disease, which creates anxiety and confusion for families [9]. Yet, such infants may go on to either develop symptoms of CF or remain healthy. Screening and sometimes confirmatory investigations provide an indication of the risk of disease [4]. In newborn screening, post-analytical tools, such as the Collaborative Laboratory Integrated Report (CLIR), are being developed to assist with such assessments of risk [10]. It may be that the outcomes of screening could be CF confirmed, CF remains possible, CF unlikely—and results communicated to families in that way.

Screening metrics are used for programme evaluation and to inform quality improvements. Whilst some programmes aim to detect all possible cases, others apply pragmatic boundaries to missed cases such as those presenting in early childhood with severe disease. It is not clear from the literature whether different programmes consider CFSPID as cases of screen-detected CF, and we think it likely that CFSPID is sometimes counted and sometimes not. Whatever approach is taken, the case definition should be clear and consistent, as it impacts screening metrics. In order to inform quality improvements, outcome data must also be available within a reasonable timeframe. The benefit of knowing about a case missed more than a decade prior is arguable given likely changes to the test methodology and algorithms in the intervening period.

2.2. Screened Population

Definitions of population screening vary but generally include a statement about screening only being appropriate for persons not at increased prior risk of having the disorder [11]. The argument for this is that at-risk infants, such as those with a family history of CF, should have genetic and functional diagnostic testing performed regardless of the newborn screen result (with genetic testing taking the particular family CFTR variants into account).

The impact of including at-risk infants in screening metrics varies depending on the screening algorithm used, and hence what is defined as a positive test.

- If the first step of the algorithm is whether family history or meconium ileus is present, and all are reported as positive screens, then all CF cases within this high-risk group will be counted as detected by screening.

- If the first step of the algorithm is to measure immunoreactive trypsin (IRT), then only those with raised IRT will be reported as screen positive, and those who have a family history but do not have raised IRT (as is common in severe disease, especially with meconium ileus detected [12]) will be counted as missed cases.
- If, following a raised IRT, the second step of the algorithm is CFTR variant analysis using a common CFTR variant panel, the screen will also miss those with family histories and a raised IRT but uncommon CFTR variants that are not included in the panel used.

2.3. Programme Boundaries

When calculating screening metrics, jurisdictions apply variable boundaries to the screening programme. Many jurisdictions only count missed cases if a normal screen result was issued. As a result, the count of missed cases is limited to those occurring within the laboratory, and due to either screening protocols or error. Whilst this definition may focus on aspects under the control of the screening laboratory, it will result in fewer missed cases and higher reported sensitivity than jurisdictions which apply a broader definition of missed cases.

CF can be missed at all steps of the screening and diagnostic pathway, including where no screening occurred or during the short-term followup [13,14]. Some jurisdictions count missed cases that occur early in the screening pathway because either the test is not offered or the family declines. Others consider the screening pathway to begin with the acceptance of a screening offer, and so would not count cases where families have declined screening because the family has effectively removed itself from the screened population. Cases may also be missed at the level of short-term followup, because the appropriate followup did not occur, or because the diagnostic test was either misinterpreted or incorrectly performed. This is particularly relevant to CF, as both methodological and biological variation can impact measured sweat chloride [15].

2.4. CF Screening Sensitivity Example

Newborn screening for CF by the measurement of IRT in dried blood spots was developed in New Zealand [1], and this was the first national programme to adopt CF screening in 1981 [16]. The programme now follows a two-step algorithm whereby samples with raised IRT (top 1%) reflex to analysis for common CFTR variants (F508del, G542X, G551D and in later years R117H). Aside from the addition of R117H, the algorithm remained the same over the period reported. The ethnic composition of New Zealand births has changed over the past decades [17] and was recently described for the period 2010–2017 [18].

Those with at least one CFTR variant are reported as positive CF screening tests. All positive tests within the Auckland region are referred to the multidisciplinary CF team at Starship Children's Hospital, who are also referred likely cases of CF from community and hospital teams within the region. We utilized the Starship Children's Hospital CF clinical database to identify new CF cases and to review CF screening in the Auckland region between 2003 and 2017.

In this time period, 325,000 babies were screened. There were 113 cases of CF diagnosed, of whom 89 were diagnosed as a result of positive newborn screening tests and 24 were clinically detected. Eight CF cases were excluded from further analysis as they had been born abroad and not screened in New Zealand. Of note, seven of these had not been screened for CF and one had a positive screen followed by a sweat test result that was considered to be normal. Table 1 outlines the relevant screening factors for the 16 New Zealand-born CF cases that were diagnosed clinically.

The calculation of screening sensitivity (the number of true positive screens divided by the sum of true positive and false negative screens, expressed as a percentage) varies depending on which clinically diagnosed CF cases are included in the count of missed cases.

- If sensitivity is calculated by counting all missed cases: 89/105 = 84.8%

- If the sensitivity calculation does not include those outside the screened population (i.e., screening declined, family history or meconium ileus) as missed cases: 89/102 = 87.3%
- If the sensitivity calculation only counts missed cases as those which occurred within the laboratory (in-range IRT, no CFTR variants on panel): 89/100 = 89.0%

Table 1. Clinically diagnosed cystic fibrosis, Auckland region 2003–2017.

	No Other Factors	Other Factors	Screening Boundary	Total
No screen			1 declined	1
In-range IRT [†]	9	1 MI [††]		10
CFTR variant not on panel	2	1 FH [†††]		3
Positive screen			2 normal sweat test	2
Total				16

[†] IRT = immunoreactive trypsin; [††] MI = meconium ileus; [†††] FH = family history.

3. Conclusions

While screening metrics are essential for both the quality assessment and improvement of programmes, they are highly dependent on the way positive tests and cases are counted. It is difficult to compare programme metrics unless definitions of the target disorder, the screened population, and the screening programme boundaries are clear and constant over time. This is particularly true for CF, where screening algorithms vary and there is a broad phenotype, as well as infants labelled with CFSPID. We suggest that in order to enable the meaningful comparison of performance data, CF screening reports should clarify what steps in the screening pathway are included in the assessment, as well as the algorithm used and screening target.

Author Contributions: Conceptualization, N.H. and D.W.; writing—original draft preparation, N.H.; writing—review and editing, D.W. All authors have read and agreed to the published version of the manuscript.

Funding: This research received no external funding.

Acknowledgments: We acknowledge the ongoing support of the National Screening Unit, Ministry of Health.

Conflicts of Interest: The authors declare no conflict of interest.

References

1. Crossley, J.R.; Elliott, R.B.; Smith, A. Dried-blood spot screening for cystic fibrosis in the newborn. *Lancet* **1979**, *1*, 472–474. [CrossRef]
2. Kerem, B.; Rommens, J.M.; Buchanan, J.A.; Markiewicz, D.; Cox, T.K.; Chakravarti, A.; Buchwald, M.; Tsui, L.C. Identification of the cystic fibrosis gene: Genetic analysis. *Science* **1989**, *245*, 1073–1080. [CrossRef] [PubMed]
3. Gilljam, M. Clinical manifestations of cystic fibrosis among patients with diagnosis in adulthood. *Chest* **2004**, *126*, 1215–1224. [CrossRef] [PubMed]
4. Pollitt, R.J. Different viewpoint: International perspectives on newborn screening. *J. Med. Biochem.* **2015**, *34*, 18–22. [CrossRef] [PubMed]
5. Farrell, P.M.; White, T.B.; Ren, C.L.; Hempstead, S.E.; Accurso, F.; Derichs, N.; Howenstine, M.; McColley, S.A.; Rock, M.; Rosenfeld, M.; et al. Diagnosis of Cystic Fibrosis: Consensus Guidelines from the Cystic Fibrosis Foundation. *J. Pediatr.* **2017**, *181S*, S4–S15.e1. [CrossRef] [PubMed]
6. Sontag, M.K.; Sarkar, D.; Comeau, A.M.; Hassell, K.; Botto, L.D.; Parad, R.; Rose, S.R.; Wintergerst, K.A.; Smith-Whitley, K.; Singh, S.; et al. Case definitions for conditions identified by newborn screening public health surveillance. *Int. J. Neonatal Screen* **2018**, *4*, 16. [CrossRef] [PubMed]
7. Munck, A.; Mayell, S.J.; Winters, V.; Shawcross, A.; Derichs, N.; Parad, R. Cystic Fibrosis Screen Positive, Inconclusive Diagnosis (CFSPID): A new designation and management recommendations for infants with an inconclusive diagnosis following newborn screening. *J. Cyst. Fibros.* **2015**, *14*, 706–713. [CrossRef] [PubMed]
8. Levy, H.; Farrell, M. New challenges in the diagnosis and management of cystic fibrosis. *J. Pediatr.* **2015**, *166*, 1337–1341. [CrossRef] [PubMed]

9. Johnson, F.; Southern, K.W.; Ulph, F. Psychological impact on parents of an inconclusive diagnosis following newborn bloodspot screening for cystic fibrosis: A qualitative study. *Int. J. Neonatal Screen* **2019**, *5*, 23. [CrossRef]
10. Collaborative Laboratory Integrated Reports. Available online: https://clir.mayo.edu (accessed on 25 May 2020).
11. National Health Committee. *Screening to Improve Health in New Zealand*; Ministry of Health: Wellington, New Zealand, 2003.
12. Sontag, M.K.; Corey, M.; Hokanson, J.E.; Marshall, J.A.; Sommer, S.S.; Zerbe, G.O.; Accurso, F.J. Genetic and physiologic correlates of longitudinal immunoreactive trypsinogen decline in infants with cystic fibrosis identified through newborn screening. *J. Pediatr.* **2006**, *149*, 650–657. [CrossRef] [PubMed]
13. Holtzman, C.; Slazyk, W.E.; Cordero, J.F.; Hannon, W.H. Descriptive epidemiology of missed cases of phenylketonuria and congenital hypothyroidism. *Pediatrics* **1986**, *78*, 553–558. [PubMed]
14. Henry, R.L.; Boulton, T.J.; Roddick, L.G. False negative results on newborn screening for cystic fibrosis. *J. Paediatr. Child Health* **1990**, *26*, 150–151. [CrossRef] [PubMed]
15. Collie, J.T.; Massie, R.J.; Jones, O.A.; LeGrys, V.A.; Greaves, R.F. Sixty-five years since the New York heat wave: Advances in sweat testing for cystic fibrosis. *Pediatr. Pulmonol.* **2014**, *49*, 106–117. [CrossRef] [PubMed]
16. Wesley, A.W.; Smith, A.; Elliott, R.B. Experience with neonatal screening for cystic fibrosis in New Zealand using measurement of immunoreactive trypsinogen. *Aust. Paediatr. J.* **1989**, *25*, 151–155. [CrossRef] [PubMed]
17. Albert, B.B.; Cutfield, W.S.; Webster, D.; Carll, J.; Derraik, J.G.B.; Jefferies, C.; Gunn, A.J.; Hofman, P.L. Etiology of increasing incidence of congenital hypothyroidism in New Zealand from 1993–2010. *J. Clin. Endocrinol. Metab.* **2012**, *97*, 3155–3160. [CrossRef] [PubMed]
18. Heather, N.L.; Derraik, J.G.; Webster, D.; Hofman, P.L. The impact of demographic factors on newborn TSH levels and congenital hypothyroidism screening. *Clin. Endocrinol. (Oxf.)* **2019**, *91*, 456–463. [CrossRef] [PubMed]

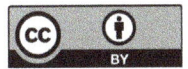

© 2020 by the authors. Licensee MDPI, Basel, Switzerland. This article is an open access article distributed under the terms and conditions of the Creative Commons Attribution (CC BY) license (http://creativecommons.org/licenses/by/4.0/).

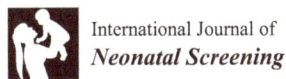

Review

Newborn Screening for CF across the Globe—*Where Is It Worthwhile*?

Virginie Scotet [1,*], Hector Gutierrez [2] and Philip M. Farrell [3]

1. Inserm, University of Brest, EFS, UMR 1078, GGB, F-29200 Brest, France
2. Department of Pediatrics, University of Alabama at Birmingham, Birmingham, AL 35233, USA; hgutierrez@peds.uab.edu
3. Departments of Pediatrics and Population Health Sciences, University of Wisconsin School of Medicine and Public Health, Madison, WI 53705, USA; pmfarrell@wisc.edu
* Correspondence: virginie.scotet@inserm.fr; Tel.: +33-298017281

Received: 31 January 2020; Accepted: 24 February 2020; Published: 4 March 2020

Abstract: Newborn screening (NBS) for cystic fibrosis (CF) has been performed in many countries for as long as four decades and has transformed the routine method for diagnosing this genetic disease and improved the quality and quantity of life for people with this potentially fatal disorder. Each region has typically undertaken CF NBS after analysis of the advantages, costs, and challenges, particularly regarding the relationship of benefits to risks. The very fact that all regions that began screening for CF have continued their programs implies that public health and clinical leaders consider early diagnosis through screening to be *worthwhile*. Currently, many regions where CF NBS has not yet been introduced are considering options and in some situations negotiating with healthcare authorities as policy and economic factors are being debated. To consider the assigned question (*where is it worthwhile*?), we have completed a worldwide analysis of data and factors that should be considered when CF NBS is being contemplated. This article describes the lessons learned from the journey toward universal screening wherever CF is prevalent and an analytical framework for application in those undecided regions. In fact, the lessons learned provide insights about what is necessary to make CF NBS *worthwhile*.

Keywords: cystic fibrosis; newborn screening; incidence; malnutrition; cost; health policy

1. Introduction

To appreciate what makes cystic fibrosis (CF) newborn screening (NBS) *worthwhile*, if not essential, it is helpful to review briefly certain historical aspects and thereby supplement the overall history described herein by Travert [1]. In particular, the perspective that follows focuses on the lessons learned about what is needed to ensure that early diagnosis through screening is indeed *worthwhile* for individuals and targeted populations. According to the Cambridge English Dictionary, *worthwhile* means "useful, important, or good enough to be a suitable reward for the money or time spent." Currently, the majority of countries in Europe and those elsewhere populated by inhabitants with European ancestry are screening newborns for CF, as shown in Figure 1. Each of these regions faced and overcame many challenges such as those listed in Table 1. Often, the combination of laboratory difficulties and complicated but necessarily efficient follow-up systems proved daunting. It may be assumed that all these regions consider CF NBS *worthwhile*. Of course, CF NBS will not prove *worthwhile* unless sustained financial support can be anticipated and all of the essential elements shown in Figure 2 are well organized and maintained. Experience has shown that the NBS system of early diagnosis and treatment requires that every step in the process be performed with assured high quality.

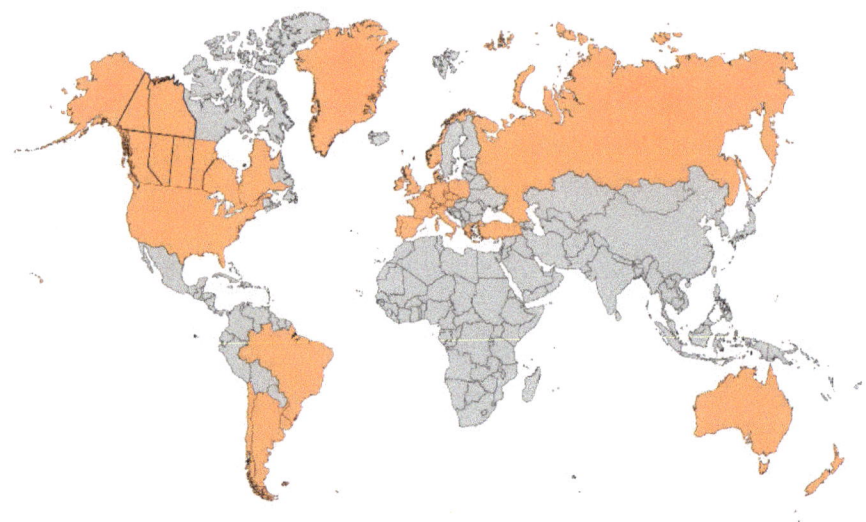

Figure 1. Worldwide implementation of cystic fibrosis newborn screening as of 2020.

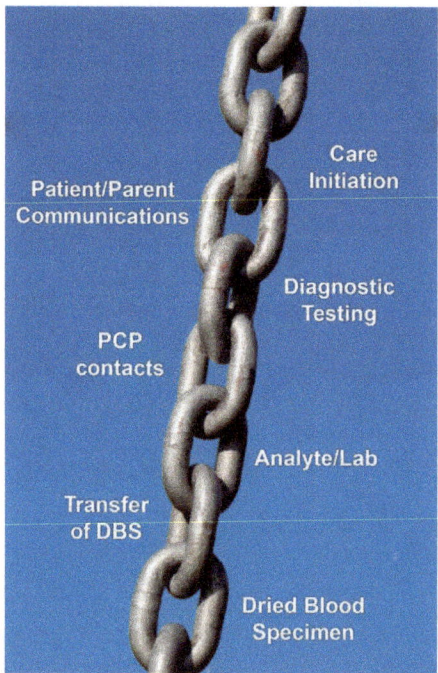

Figure 2. The sequence of processes and procedures linked together like a chain in the system of early diagnosis via newborn screening, reminding us that "a chain is only as strong as its weakest link." Abbreviations include PCP—primary care provider; DBS—dried blood specimen.

Table 1. Essential elements to ensure that cystic fibrosis newborn screening is *worthwhile*.

1	A system must be established and functioning well for the universal collection of dried blood spot specimens and their analysis in a central laboratory with quality assurance mechanisms in place and a goal to maximum sensitivity with acceptable specificity.
2	Collaborative efforts by a team that includes NBS laboratory leadership and CF center follow-up clinicians organized to operate efficiently.
3	Effective CF NBS analytical tests organized as a sequential protocol (algorithm) to maximize sensitivity and optimize specificity.
4	Quality improvements in laboratory methods must be planned for and implemented as technologies advance rather than accepting the *status quo* and resisting change.
5	Expeditious follow-up care must ensure that not only will high-quality sweat testing be provided promptly to confirm diagnoses but that the nutritional benefits are achieved immediately by a team of dedicated, experienced caregivers with gastrointestinal/nutritional expertise.
6	A cohort follow-up system must be ensured for patients diagnosed as neonates to segregate them from older patients and avoid exposure to virulent respiratory pathogens.
7	To ensure a favorable benefit: risk relationship, preventive management of potential psychosocial harms must be given priority by a skilled, dedicated follow-up team.
8	The incidence of CF must be high enough to warrant CF care centers in the NBS region.
9	The NBS system must be organized as a highly efficient operation that avoids preventable delays and ensures consistently diagnostic timeliness.
10	CF NBS guidelines should be known and adhered to throughout the sequence of integrated processes.

2. Requirements That Must Be Met for CF NBS to Be *Worthwhile*

2.1. Feasibility of Screening Newborns for CF

The requirements that must be addressed to implement and maintain a successful NBS program for CF are listed in Table 1. Although attempts to achieve early diagnosis of CF through meconium tests were organized during the 1970s [2], NBS first became feasible on a population scale in 1979 when dried blood spots were analyzed for immunoreactive trypsinogen (IRT) in New Zealand by Crossley et al. [3]. Through retrospective assessment, they found that high IRT levels revealed a significant risk for CF. The utility and convenience of dried blood spots in NBS had, of course, been obvious since their application in 1963 to phenylketonuria [4], and many public health laboratories worldwide were already screening for hereditary metabolic disorders and congenital endocrinopathies. Thus, the first requirement for the *worthwhile* implementation of CF NBS is to have a system in place and functioning well for the universal collection of dried blood spot specimens and their analysis in a central laboratory with quality assurance mechanisms in place. The seminal research in New Zealand was only possible because the NBS laboratory there collaborated closely with the University of Auckland Paediatrics Department across the street. The lesson learned there has been demonstrated repeatedly, namely that to be *worthwhile*, CF NBS must be a collaborative effort with a dedicated team that addresses every component of the sequence shown in Figure 2. For those few engaged in CF NBS using meconium tests in the 1970s, the report of Crossley et al. [3] had an immediate, profound influence, stimulating research around the world. On the other hand, the availability of a screening test alone is insufficient to justify its implementation as Wilson and Jungner [5] emphasized five decades ago.

2.2. The Need for an Excellent Screening Test: Limitations of IRT/IRT

The breakthrough discovery in New Zealand was followed by important studies in New South Wales in Australia [6], Colorado [7], and France [8]. Leaders in each of these regions recognized the potential benefits of early diagnosis ranging from epidemiologic and clinical research opportunities to care enhancement and improvement in the organization of healthcare delivery. Much skepticism remained, however, because of concerns about the IRT test per se, whether or not significant clinical benefits actually occurred, and how much adverse impact was being imposed on parents of screened neonates, i.e., the degree of psychosocial harm. In retrospect, the major concern that limited CF NBS acceptance, and thus a third lesson learned, concerns the IRT/IRT screening strategy—a method with relatively low sensitivity that requires a second, confirming blood specimen at approximately two weeks of age. Consequently, this first phase of experience with dried blood spot screening led to a realization that more research was needed on all aspects of CF NBS and the IRT method of screening needed to be improved. In fact, a decade after the report from New Zealand there was worldwide debate among health policy decision-makers whether or not CF NBS was *worthwhile* and even doubt among organizations like the U.S. Cystic Fibrosis Foundation—expressed emphatically when it sponsored a negative but influential commentary [9]. Consequently, CF NBS implementation was slow in North America and Europe, and one country (France) even discontinued their national IRT-based program.

2.3. The Value of the IRT/DNA Screening Test When CFTR Mutations Are Known

The view that IRT/IRT was not sufficiently sensitive with practical cutoff values coupled to the discovery of the *CFTR* gene in 1989 [10] and its principal disease-causing variant, p.Phe508del (F508del), led almost immediately to a search for a better screening algorithm in some regions. Others, however, continued IRT/IRT and either tolerated, or did not recognize, its relatively low sensitivity of 75–80% [11]. In retrospect, the discovery that about 90% of Europeans and Europe-derived CF populations have at least one p.Phe508del variant greatly facilitated the development of the first DNA-based NBS test, the IRT/DNA(p.Phe508del) method [12]. Soon thereafter, the DNA tier was expanded to a *CFTR* multimutation panel and a sensitivity of >95% was achieved routinely [13]. In addition, the quality of screening improved significantly by allowing test completion on the initial dried blood spot specimen, thus improving timeliness, and by providing valuable information on *CFTR* mutations. It was quickly learned with IRT/DNA(*CFTR*) that the vast majority of CF cases can be presumptively (genetically) diagnosed within a week of birth from the initial blood specimen and valuable genetic data obtained to predict pancreatic functional status.

The lesson learned from these experiences is clear: although initiating CF NBS with the IRT biomarker alone is much better than no screening for CF, regions should plan from the outset on improving their laboratory methods, ideally with a DNA-based second-tier method as *CFTR* population data emerge and enable transformation to a better, DNA-based algorithm that can make CF NBS more *worthwhile*. Another alternative is to use pancreatitis-associated protein (PAP) as an adjunct but a variety of issues limit its effectiveness [14]. The motivation for including PAP as a secondary biomarker in the screening strategy was to limit the incidental findings inherent to the use of DNA analysis such as the detection of carriers and the recognition of equivocal clinical phenotypes [14]. With any algorithm, tracking and evaluating data annually is an essential component of monitoring screening outcome measures such as sensitivity, specificity, positive predictive value, age of diagnosis to ensure that timeliness is achieved and disease incidence.

2.4. The Challenge of Evaluating and Achieving Benefits That Outweigh Risks

No NBS test has been subjected to more skepticism or scrutiny than CF screening even when the unique value of the IRT/DNA screening became evident. The rationale illustrated in Figure 3 has been considered so intuitive for other genetic conditions that implementation with little or no clinical evidence is typical for most screening tests and cost-effectiveness is generally not assessed. In retrospect, the debates in the CF community that raged over whether or not actual benefits occur and, if so, the benefit: risk relationship seems surprising when the potentially fatal salt loss in sweat and protein-energy malnutrition are well known to have plagued children with CF for decades [15]. Thus, the proof was demanded for the efficacy of CF NBS. However, the very short pre-symptomatic phase of CF, illustrated in Figure 3, was not appreciated until studies of infants diagnosed through NBS were published and revealed that malnutrition may occur within days and lung disease within weeks [15].

Eventually, convincing results from organized trials in Wales [16], Wisconsin [17], and elsewhere were published and confirmed, along with other supportive data on benefits [18]. The Wisconsin study, a randomized clinical trial assessing 650,341 infants during nine years of enrollment demonstrated short- and long-term nutritional benefits with early, aggressive care management [19,20] and less lung disease in those responding well to better nutrition [21].

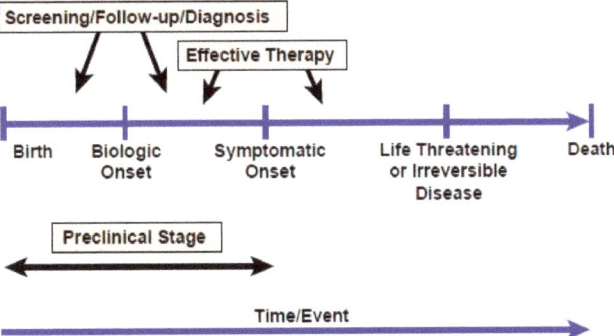

Figure 3. The rationale for early diagnosis via newborn screening by applying the principle inherent in the preventive medicine strategy to detect disease before its symptomatic onset.

In retrospect, it is much easier to evaluate nutritional outcomes after NBS than the course of lung disease, particularly in children, because of the numerous variables influencing the respiratory system as illustrated in Figure 4, including environmental factors such as respiratory pathogen exposures that are difficult to quantitate. The lesson learned from this experience is that for CF NBS to be *worthwhile*, expeditious follow-up care must ensure that not only will high-quality sweat testing be provided promptly to confirm diagnoses but that the nutritional benefits are achieved immediately by a team of dedicated, experienced caregivers with gastrointestinal/nutritional expertise. Thus, regional data tracking methods should assess multiple indices of nutritional status and monitor growth velocity carefully during the first two years of life. If growth failure occurs, comprehensive assessments and more aggressive nutritional interventions are essential, but more research is needed on supplements such as essential fatty acids.

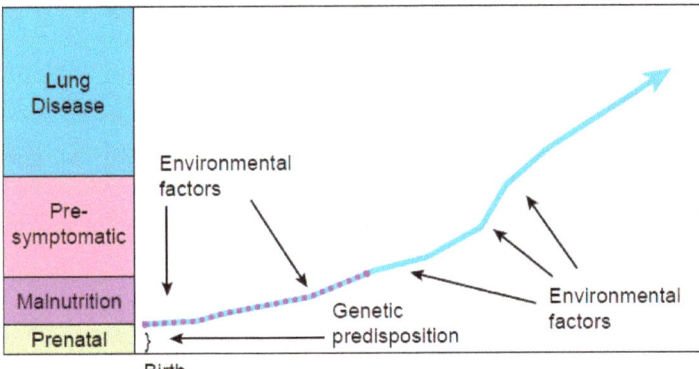

Figure 4. The many intrinsic and extrinsic variables (risk factors) that influence the course of cystic fibrosis and have much more impact on lung disease over a longer time period than those that affect nutritional status. The numerous environmental factors include exposures to smoke, virulent respiratory bacterial pathogens such as mucoid *Pseudomonas aeruginosa*, respiratory virus epidemics, etc.

Management of the respiratory complications of CF after NBS is more challenging with conventional therapies. Early diagnosis provides the opportunity to initiate some prophylactic measures, monitor for signs and symptoms of lung disease, and intervene quickly. A lesson learned in the Wisconsin trial is that infants must be segregated from older patients to avoid exposure to virulent respiratory pathogens [22]. Although cohorting non-infected patients was not the standard practice during the 20th century, this preventive strategy is essential to make CF NBS *worthwhile* [23,24]. Thus, regions contemplating the initiation of a screening program need to organize a segregated follow-up system for patients diagnosed as neonates. In addition, if/when more CFTR modulator therapy options become approved for infants with the p.Phe508del variant and routine organ preservation a routine reality, all regions will need to ensure the availability of these expensive therapies. In addition, access to care and avoidance of disparities needs to be assured.

With regard to the risks of CF NBS, many investigations worldwide have focused on potential psychosocial harms [25,26], especially in false-positive families, but it should be recognized that these risks accompany every screening test whether infants or older individuals are being screened. However, some have argued that CF NBS deserves more attention than that given to other conditions, and certainly there have been more studies on the potential risks. Recognizing the importance of the benefit: risk relationship, the Wisconsin team conducted their trial as a comprehensive longitudinal project that assessed adverse outcome potential through a variety of psychosocial studies and interviews [27,28]. The advantages and challenges of genetic counseling were also investigated and generally shown to be beneficial [29]. In summary, the lesson learned is that psychosocial harms may indeed occur, primarily due to misunderstanding of test results and their implications, but that investment by the follow-up team in proactive, excellent communication efforts can prevent and/or alleviate this risk which applies particularly to families experiencing false-positive tests. The importance of such tactics is underscored when a baby is identified as having CRMS/CFSPID (cystic fibrosis transmembrane conductance regulator-related metabolic syndrome/cystic fibrosis screen positive, inconclusive diagnosis) [30]. This condition is considered a "byproduct" of CF NBS with the IRT tier and often presents a diagnostic dilemma. In these cases, and whenever CF is diagnosed, genetic counseling is essential and should be an integral part of the follow-up efforts [29].

3. Criteria to Implement Screening

3.1. European CF Society Guidelines

The European Cystic Fibrosis Society (ECFS) has published best practice guidelines for CF NBS [31] that are applicable to the question *Where is it worthwhile?* These deal with population characteristics such as the incidence of CF in a given region, the health and social support resources that are "minimally acceptable for newborn screening to be a valid undertaking," the quality of dried blood samples, acceptable levels of sensitivity and specificity, and the importance of timeliness. Table 2 summarizes the ECFS recommendations.

We respectfully disagree with the view that an incidence of at least 1:7000 hould guide decisions about whether or not to screen. In fact, many genetic disorders included in standard NBS panels have a much lower incidence without any challenge to their validity [32]. Many of the hereditary metabolic disorders in NBS panels have incidences of 1:200,000–3,000,000, as David et al. [32] emphasize. In addition, with CF NBS underway for extensive periods, the incidence of CF may decrease significantly [33] and even in previously high incidence regions become less than 1:7000. Certainly, these regions should not discontinue their programs. In view of the wide range of CF incidence data in countries with sufficient CF prevalence to warrant CF care centers and the reduction potential of prenatal and neonatal screening, we are reluctant to specify an incidence criterion; however, based on the typical panel of hereditary metabolic diseases in current screening programs of the western world, greater than 1:25,000 would be reasonable. It should be emphasized that the criteria established by Wilson and Jungner in 1968 [5] for the implementation of a screening program in the general population did not include the concept of a minimal incidence.

Table 2. European Cystic Fibrosis Society (ECFS) best practice guidelines: the 2018 revision [31].

1	Population characteristics that validate screening newborn infants for CF."Health authorities need to balance the benefit/risk ratio of screening newborns for CF in their population. If the incidence of CF is <1/7000 births, careful evaluation is required as to whether NBS is valid. The protocol must be shown to cause the minimum negative impact possible on the population. Other factors in making the decision on whether to implement screening should include available healthcare resources and the ability to provide a clear pathway to treatment."
2	Health and social resources that are minimally acceptable for NBS to be a valid undertaking."Infants identified with CF through a NBS program should have prompt access to specialist CF care that achieves ECFS standards. A NBS program may be a mechanism to better organize CF services, through the direct referral of infants for specialist CF care. Countries with limited resources should consider a pilot study to assess the validity of NBS and the adequacy of referral services for newly diagnosed infants in their population."
3	Acceptable number of repeat tests required for inadequate dried blood samples for every 1000 infants screened."The number of requests for repeat dried blood samples should be monitored and should be 0.5%. More than 20 repeats for every 1000 infants, is unacceptable (2%)."
4	Acceptable number of false-positive NBS results (infants referred for clinical assessment and sweat testing)."Programmes should aim for a minimum positive predictive value of 0.3 (PPV is the number of infants with a true positive NBS test divided by the total number of positive NBS tests)."
5	Acceptable number of false-negative NBS results. These are infants with a negative NBS test that are subsequently diagnosed with CF (a delayed diagnosis)."Programmes should aim for a minimum sensitivity of 95%."
6	Maximum acceptable delay between a sweat test being undertaken and the result given to the family. "The sweat test should be analyzed immediately and the result reported to the family on the same day."
7	Maximum acceptable age of an infant on the day they are first reviewed by a specialist CF team following a diagnosis of CF after NBS."The majority of infants with a confirmed diagnosis after NBS should be seen by a specialist CF team by 35 days and no later than 58 days after birth."
8	Minimum acceptable information for families of an infant recognized to be a carrier of a CF-causing mutation after NBS.Families should receive a verbal report of the result. They should also receive written information to refer to. Information should also be sent to the family Primary Care Physician. The information should be clear that the infant does not have CF; the baby is a healthy carrier; future pregnancies for this couple are not free of risk of CF and the parents may opt for genetic counseling, and there are implications that could affect reproductive decision making for extended family members and the infant when they are of childbearing age.

The ECFS recommendation that "programmes should aim for a minimum sensitivity of 95%" is appropriate but unattainable in regions using IRT/IRT or some other combination of biomarkers. Such regions are often limited by inadequate knowledge of the *CFTR* mutations prevalent in their population, but as that information is gained transformation to a more sensitive screening test can be accomplished.

The issue of follow-up efficiency was also addressed in the ECFS guidelines. First, it is stated that a sweat test result should be completed and the result reported to the family on the same day—an ideal practice but unfortunately not always routinely done. With regard to timeliness, the guidelines recommend 35–58 days after birth for the "maximum acceptable age of an infant on the day they are first reviewed by a special CF team following a diagnosis of CF after NBS." This recommendation was influenced by practical considerations in various European countries, but undoubtedly infants with CF are susceptible to potentially fatal salt loss in sweat prior to the 35–58-day interval, especially in hot climates and with breastfeeding. In addition, CF infants certainly can develop biochemically severe nutritional abnormalities within 2–4 weeks of birth and even suffer the onset of lung disease within 1–2 months. In addition, the recent data suggesting that organ preservation can be achieved with early CFTR modulator therapy [34] argues for diagnosis as soon after birth as possible. Consequently, a more efficient plan promulgated by some organizations recommends diagnosis as early as 2 weeks of age and definitely by 4 weeks of age. To be *worthwhile*, therefore, regions should organize their CF NBS programs to be highly efficient and avoid any preventable delays.

3.2. Clinical and Laboratory Standards Institute, the Association of Public Health Laboratories, the Centers for Disease Control and Prevention, and the Cystic Fibrosis Foundation

In the United States, the group of organizations listed above has worked collaboratively in the area of CF NBS to ensure expeditious nationwide implementation and ongoing attention to quality improvement. The CLSI recently published new guidelines [35] to revise the recommendations of 2011 focusing on the six aspects of CF NBS listed below as the responsible Document Development Committee identified the key areas of quality improvement.

(1) Reassessed IRT cutoff value guidelines and discussed the use of a floating rather than fixed cutoff value. The floating cutoff strategy using the 95th or 96th percentile helps overcome the seasonal and kit-related variations in IRT [11]. The recommendations included: "Recent data have shown that the traditional IRT cutoff values in the IRT/IRT algorithm were too high to minimize false-negative screening results and the 95th to 97th percentile (approximately 60 ng/mL) should be used." As expanded genetic analyses and next-generation sequencing are becoming less expensive, some CF NBS programs are operating with a lower fixed IRT (for example 40 ng/mL), thus allowing more samples for genetic testing to reduce false-negative screening results.

(2) Revised recommendations regarding *CFTR* variant panels based on the most current information including new biotechnologies such as next-generation sequencing, pointing out that "Guidelines published in 2001 and revised in 2004 include recommendations for screening with a *CFTR* variant panel of 23 disease-causing variants with a prevalence of at least 0.1% in the CF population. Although this recommended panel provides a high CF detection rate... additional variants may need to be added for improved CF detection in other ethnic groups. Many NBS programs use larger *CFTR* variant panels..."

(3) Assessed using PAP for detecting babies at risk for CF but did not make a recommendation.

(4) Discussed communications strategies related to the detecting of CF heterozygote babies and providing genetic counseling.

(5) Reviewed emerging issues related to using genetic and genomic sequencing in NBS.

(6) Described the existing CF NBS algorithms, while commenting on the advantages and disadvantages of each protocol.

The U.S. CF Foundation organized a recent diagnosis consensus with international input to (1) clarify the criteria that need to be met for diagnosis via either NBS or after signs/symptoms; (2) emphasize the importance of efficient follow-up of positive screening tests; (3) describe how to apply and communicate genetic data; (4) harmonize the definition of CRMS and CFSPID [36]. These guidelines recommend that sweat testing be performed as soon as possible after 10 days of age, ideally by 28 days of age. They also point out that treatment should not be delayed when sweat testing is unsuccessful. The Association of Public Health Laboratories, through its NewSTEPs program, has also emphasized timeliness. Lastly, the Centers for Disease Control and Prevention has established an invaluable quality assurance monitoring program for worldwide assistance *gratis* and a molecular assessment program, which conducts site visits to U.S. NBS laboratories that carry out molecular testing.

For CF NBS to be *worthwhile*, all the guidelines and recommendations summarized above should be well known to the leaders of screening regions and those that wish to implement programs. In the past, too many regions initiated CF NBS programs without taking advantage of the readily available resources and experience of established programs.

Int. J. Neonatal Screen. **2020**, *6*, 18

4. Incidence of CF around the World and Screening Protocols Being Employed

Figures 5 and 6 provide data on the estimated incidence of CF in many regions. Through a complete registration of cases directly at birth, the implementation of CF NBS has allowed a more accurate determination of the incidence of CF and better monitoring of its time trends. Before the implementation of NBS, the incidence estimation was mainly based on epidemiological studies that generally suffered from ascertainment bias due to under-diagnosis and/or under-reporting of cases. However, with NBS data, care must be taken when interpreting incidence data, as variations may occur depending on the patients included in the calculations (e.g., false-negatives, patients with meconium ileus, patients with CFSPID). In order to have consistent data, it is important to ensure that the calculations are based on the same population. The incidence data may also be biased by a short observation period in some studies.

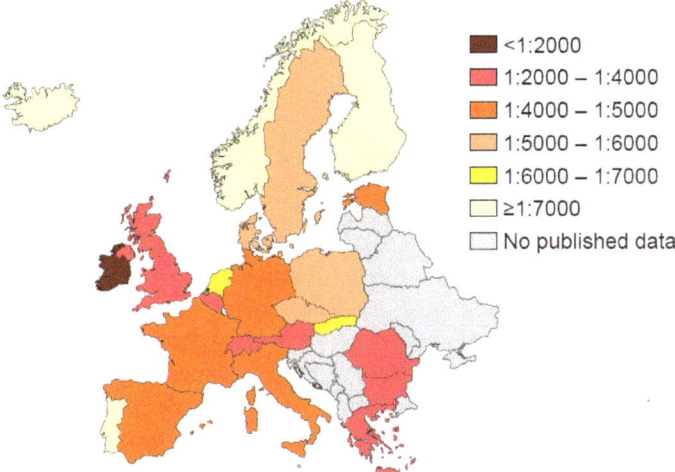

Figure 5. Incidence of cystic fibrosis in Europe.

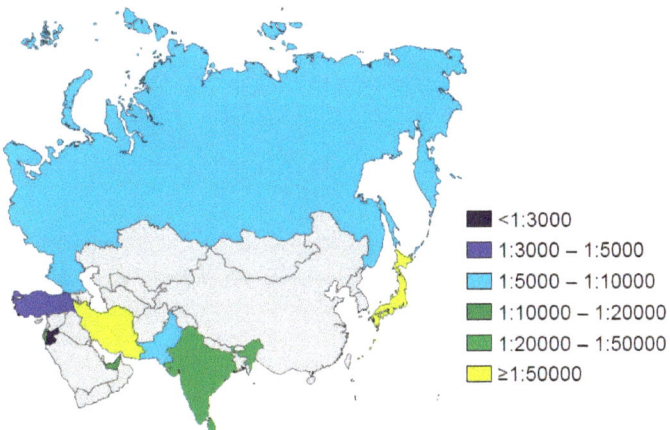

Figure 6. Incidence of cystic fibrosis in Asia.

4.1. Europe

The incidence of CF has long been estimated at 1:2500 in the European population [37]. In 2007, a review of CF NBS programs revealed that the incidence was on average 1:3500 [38] and it appears still lower nowadays. Beyond Ireland which has the highest incidence of CF in Europe (1:1353) [39], the incidence ranges from 1:2800 in the UK [38] to 1:10,000 in Russia [40] (Figure 5). It is 1:2850 in Belgium [41], about 1:4500 in France [42], Germany [14], Italy [38,43,44], and Spain (where large regional variations are observed) [45], while it oscillates between 1:5200 and 1:6500 in Central Europe (Czech Republic [32], Denmark [46], Netherlands [47], Poland [48], Slovakia [49], and Sweden [50]). The incidence appears lower than 1:7000 in three European countries (Portugal [51], Norway [52], and Russia [40]) as well as in various regions of Spain [45]. In countries without NBS, the incidence ranges from 1:2000 (Romania [53]) to 1:25,000 (Finland [54]).

The implementation of CF NBS across Europe has gradually spread, with a faster pace during the past decade. From the update performed by Barben et al. in 2016 [55] and the data acquired since, CF NBS has been implemented in 22 European countries to date (Figure 7). Nineteen countries have a national program and three have regional programs (which cover the whole country for Spain). The number of countries with a national NBS program has gradually increased over the past years, from 2 in 2007 (France and Austria) to 19 to date. Twenty-four countries have no NBS program but nine are considering or planning to implement screening protocols. The screening protocols, however, are varied and all national programs have a distinct algorithm. As illustrated in Figure 7, most programs use DNA analysis as a second-tier test, while five (Austria, Portugal, Russia, Slovakia, and Turkey) still rely exclusively on biochemical tests. The expansion of CF NBS across Europe has been successful and reveals that this screening is considered *worthwhile*.

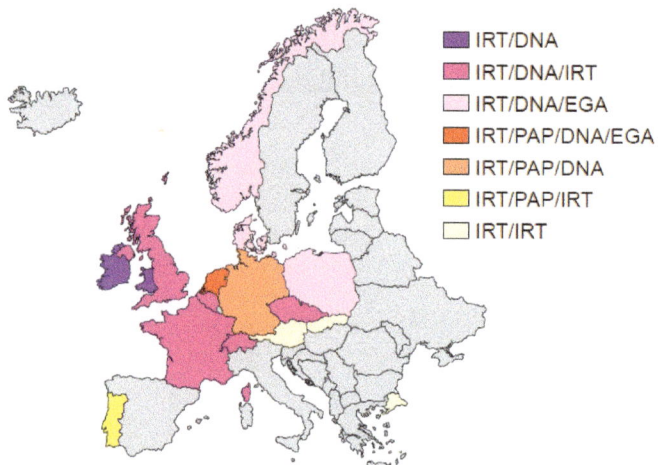

Figure 7. Protocols used in newborn screening for cystic fibrosis in Europe in 2020. Abbreviations include IRT—immunoreactive trypsinogen; EGA—expanded or extended gene analysis; PAP—pancreatitis-associated protein.

4.2. Australasia

The incidence of CF is well defined in Australasia as CF NBS has been in place for a very long time in this part of Oceania. The incidence is approximately 1:3000. It has been estimated as 1:2821 in New South Wales [56], 1:3139 in Victoria [57], and 1:3180 in New Zealand [58]. Newborn screening for CF has been performed for almost 40 years (1981) in New Zealand—which was the first country to implement a national program (1981) and for almost 20 years in all states within Australia where CF

NBS was first introduced in New South Wales during 1981 [56]. Currently, all states use a DNA-based NBS program. The very long experience of Australasia in CF NBS confirms the view that is this screening is deemed *worthwhile* in that part of the world.

4.3. United States of America

The incidence of CF for the entire population is approximately 1:4000, but ethnicity-related variations occur and have a regional impact [59]. In the white population, about 1 in 3000 babies are at risk for CF. Although limited data have been collected and analyzed on "minority" populations, it appears that the incidence and Hispanic infants are about 1:6000 and in African-Americans at least 1:10,000. Disparities in the age of diagnosis and ascertainment of CF cases may occur in these "minority" populations, so more data are needed. It has become increasingly clear that *CFTR* panels need to be expanded to reduce disparities, but NBS labs in the U.S. are notoriously slow to change methodologies as evidenced by a 10-year delay in all states transforming from IRT/IRT to IRT/DNA or IRT/IRT/DNA protocols after unequivocal evidence was published [11]. However, during the current year, all states are using DNA-based CF NBS and all consider their programs *worthwhile*.

4.4. Canada

The incidence of CF has been well defined during the past decade in Canada as all 10 provinces implemented CF NBS from 2007, beginning with Alberta, to 2017 when Québec implemented their excellent program based on clinical outcomes. In general, the Canadian population is more Euro-American than in other American countries. Therefore, it is not surprising that the incidence of CF is higher—averaging about 1:3300 [60]. Moreover, Québec in its first two years of CF NBS identified a 1:2300 incidence. The relatively high prevalence of CF throughout Canada and the excellent CF care centers providing follow-up and early treatment have certainly made CF NBS *worthwhile* there using DNA-based protocols.

4.5. Latin America—Mexico (North America), Central, and South America

The Latin American population is one of the most diverse in the world, due to a variety of ancestries, ethnicities, and races that have mixed for centuries. The dominant racial groups in the region are Caucasians, European-Amerindian (mestizo), Black, and Amerindian. The proportion of each group varies significantly among the Latin American countries [61]. Given this complex composition, the incidence of CF is difficult to foretell and is further complicated because many countries lack established clinical programs, newborn screening, and registries.

The racial distribution of CF cases, as illustrated by the 2017 Brazilian Registry, highlights the diversity of CF in Latin America. Of 5128 cases, 68% are white (branca), 25% are mestizo (parda), and 6% are black (preta). There are just a small number of cases of Asian (amarela) and Amerindian (indigena) descent.

Of 29,887 patients reported by the U.S. Cystic Fibrosis Foundation Patient Registry 2017 Annual Data Report, 8.7% are Hispanics. Extrapolating the current prevalence of CF in the US Hispanic population to Latin America, one could expect about 30,000 people with CF in the region. It should be pointed out that most of the Hispanics in the U.S. come from Mexico and Central America, which has a lower proportion of people of European descent that countries like Argentina, Uruguay, Chile, and Brazil [62]. Thus, the above prevalence might underestimate the number of people with CF.

Currently, reliable data on the incidence of CF in Latin America is lacking, in part, due to limited diagnostic accuracy. There is no neonatal screening in most of the countries, and genetic panels have a low diagnostic yield because they do not reflect the ethnic admixture of the population [63].

4.5.1. Argentina

Although Argentina approved legislation for mandatory administration of neonatal screening for CF in 1994, it has never reached meaningful national coverage (15%–20%). A recent report from the Grupo Registro Nacional de Fibrosis Quistica (National CF Registry Taskforce), verified that the neonatal screening in 2012 had coverage of 28.8%. The CF National Consensus of 2008 reported that between 1995 and 2005, CF incidence was 1:6131, after screening almost 1 million infants. There is no defined protocol for its performance. The most commonly used is IRT/IRT. The Autonomous City of Buenos Aires (CABA) started its neonatal screening in 2002, using the IRT/IRT algorithm. From 2002–2014, the incidence was 1:7444 (49/364,782; V. Rodriguez, personal communication). In 2015, Buenos Aires modified the algorithm to IRT/PAP.

4.5.2. Brazil

Brazil has developed the most robust CF care structure, similar to the OECD countries, including a CF center network, sophisticated registry, and neonatal screening. Adoption of the neonatal screening (IRT/IRT) has gained prominence in diagnosing new cases, from 32% in 2009 to 61% in 2017. The reported incidence varies among different states, higher in the South Region (Santa Catarina: 1:6500; Paraná: 1:9000), lower in others (Minas Gerais: 1:11,000), (V. Rodriguez, personal communication).

4.5.3. Chile

Studies from the mid-1990s reported an incidence of 1:4000 (Rios, 1994). More recent data from two pilot studies on neonatal screening puts the incidence between 1:8000 and 1:10,000 (2015–2017; ML Boza, personal communication). Chile anticipates starting national CF neonatal screening in 2020, using the IRT/PAP protocol.

4.5.4. Mexico

There is no accurate data on incidence. In 2016, the Secretaria de Salud (Ministry of Health) reported 350 new cases of CF per year. Averaging 2.3 million births per year over the last decade, Mexico could have an incidence of approximately 1:6700. Others have reported a lower rate (1:8500; 2002, Jose Luis Lezana, personal communication). Neonatal screening for CF was added to the national program in 2015. The screening method currently used is IRT/IRT. As it has been the norm in the Latin American countries, the use of mutation panels has low yields (A 34-mutation panel had a sensitivity of <75%; Orozco, 2000).

4.5.5. Uruguay

Uruguay implemented neonatal screening in 2010. Initially using the IRT/IRT protocol, but changing to IRT/PAP in 2012. Analysis from years 2010– 2016 totaling 322,727 screened babies, 39 confirmed diagnoses, puts the incidence in 1:8300 (C Pinchack, personal communication).

4.5.6. Other Latin American Countries

In 2019 Colombia and Peru approved the addition of CF screening into their national newborn screenings. We have no information on the protocols used. Also, the incidence in these countries has not been established. Costa Rica has had CF neonatal screening for several years but has not reached full coverage. Seven cases on average per year suggest an incidence of 1:15,000 (J. Gutierrez, personal communication). An ongoing pilot study puts the rate in 1:10,000.

4.5.7. Is CF Neonatal Screening *Worthwhile* in Latin American Countries?

With an expected high number of cases and the late age in diagnosis that presently occurs, the use of neonatal screening should be a cost-effective tool to help to identify patients at a younger age, therefore improving survival.

4.6. Asia

Although the incidence of CF in Asia has long been unknown, the existence of CF in that continent is now well established. The incidence is greatly variable and appears much higher in the Middle East than in East Asia (Figure 6). Cases of CF have been reported in many Arab countries and in some of them (where consanguinity is common), the incidence appears close to that observed in populations of European descent. It has thus been estimated to 1:2560 in Jordan [64] or to 1:5800 in Bahrain [65], while it is about 1:16,000 in the United Arab Emirates [66] and in Israel, where the incidence has dropped significantly following implementation of population carrier screening program [67]. The incidence of CF is lower in South Asian populations. It has been estimated between 1:10,000 and 1:100,000 in the Indian population [68–71] and to 1:90,000 in an Oriental population living in Hawaii [72]. The incidence is very low in Japan (1:350,000) [73] as well as in China where less than 30 cases have been reported over the two last decades [74]. Thus, CF NBS would not seem *worthwhile* in those countries.

Beyond variability in carrier frequency, the wide range observed in incidence may be in part explained by under-diagnosis and under-reporting of cases [75,76]. The incidence of CF in Asia may therefore be under-estimated. Despite the low incidence of CF in that continent, the number of CF patients must be high in some countries due to the large population size (such as India).

In Arab countries, the major challenges are to improve the diagnosis and the detection of mutations before irreversible organ damage has developed and to promote the constitution of national registries [75,76], which will help to improve CF management and health policy planning. To the best of our knowledge, no CF NBS program is implemented to date in the Arab world, but CF NBS is promoted by the annual meeting for NBS in the Middle East and North Africa. The sole country that was considering implementing an NBS program during 2020 is Israel.

In view of the high incidence of CF in some Arab countries and the genomic revolution that is underway in those countries (through the Saudi, Qatar, and Emirati genome projects), CF NBS should be *worthwhile* in the regions where CF is well managed. NBS programs would have to take into account the genetic specificities of that population (limited mutation spectrum, lower prevalence of p.Phe508del mutation, mutations found only in that population [76]) but also the high consanguinity rate.

5. Summary

Newborn screening for CF has been performed in many countries for as long as four decades and has transformed the routine method for diagnosing this genetic disease and improved the quality and quantity of life for people with this potentially fatal disorder. Each region has typically undertaken CF NBS after analysis of the advantages, costs, and challenges, particularly regarding the relationship of benefits to risks. The very fact that all regions that began screening for CF have continued their programs implies that public health and clinical leaders consider early diagnosis through screening to be *worthwhile*. In this article, after summarizing the considerations that led the majority of North American and European countries to implement CF NBS programs successfully, we analyze countries that are or should be planning to screen newborns for this relatively common genetic disorder. From this analysis, we suggest the criteria listed in Table 3. Recent, dramatic advances in therapies offer great promise for all patients diagnosed early and especially children diagnosed before pathology quickly develops irreversibly.

Table 3. Suggested criteria for cystic fibrosis newborn screening.

Incidence of CF: greater than 1:25,000
Aim at minimum sensitivity of 95%
IRT/DNA—unless unavailable or not feasible
Diagnosis including sweat chloride within 4 weeks of age
Assessment program for tests, including plans for monitoring and updating
Availability of a complete specialist CF team

Author Contributions: All authors participated in conceptualization, writing the original draft, and devoting efforts to review and editing work. V.S. was responsible for submitting the manuscript and reviewing/correcting the proofs. All authors have read and agreed to the published version of the manuscript.

Funding: V.S. is supported by Inserm; P.M.F. and H.G. are supported by the U.S. Cystic Fibrosis Foundation.

Acknowledgments: The authors thank Robert Gordon of the Department of Pediatrics at the University of Wisconsin School of Medicine and Public Health for his superb computer graphics efforts to create the illustrations published herein. They also thank Jürg Barben, Kevin Southern, and Anne Munck for providing updated data on newborn screening for cystic fibrosis in Europe.

Conflicts of Interest: The authors declare no conflict of interest.

References

1. Travert, G.; Heeley, M.; Heeley, A. History of newborn screening for CF—The Early Years. *Int. J. Neonatal Screen.* **2020**, *6*, 8. [CrossRef]
2. Bruns, W.T.; Connell, T.R.; Lacey, J.A.; Whisler, K.E. Test strip meconium screening for cystic fibrosis. *Am. J. Dis. Child.* **1977**, *131*, 71–73. [CrossRef] [PubMed]
3. Crossley, J.R.; Elliott, R.B.; Smith, P.A. Dried-blood spot screening for cystic fibrosis in the newborn. *Lancet* **1979**, *1*, 472–474. [CrossRef]
4. Guthrie, R.; Susi, A. A Simple Phenylalanine Method for Detecting Phenylketonuria in Large Populations of Newborn Infants. *Pediatrics* **1963**, *32*, 338–343.
5. Wilson, J.M.G.; Jungner, Y.G. *Principles and Practice of Screening for Disease*; WHO: Geneva, Switzerland, 1968; Available online: http://www.who.int/bulletin/volumes/86/4/07-050112BP.pdf (accessed on 1 March 2020).
6. Wilcken, B.; Brown, A.R.; Urwin, R.; Brown, D.A. Cystic fibrosis screening by dried blood spot trypsin assay: Results in 75,000 newborn infants. *J. Pediatr.* **1983**, *102*, 383–387. [CrossRef]
7. Reardon, M.C.; Hammond, K.B.; Accurso, F.J.; Fisher, C.D.; McCabe, E.R.; Cotton, E.K.; Bowman, C.M. Nutritional deficits exist before 2 months of age in some infants with cystic fibrosis identified by screening test. *J. Pediatr.* **1984**, *105*, 271–274. [CrossRef]
8. Travert, G.; Duhamel, J.F. Systematic neonatal screening for mucoviscidosis using an immunoreactive trypsin blood assay. Evaluation of 80,000 tests. *Arch. Fr. Pediatr.* **1983**, *40*, 295–298.
9. Cystic Fibrosis Foundation, Ad Hoc Committee Task Force on Neonatal Screening. Neonatal screening for cystic fibrosis: Position paper. *Pediatrics* **1983**, *72*, 741–745.
10. Kerem, B.; Rommens, J.M.; Buchanan, J.A.; Markiewicz, D.; Cox, T.K.; Chakravarti, A.; Buchwald, M.; Tsui, L.C. Identification of the cystic fibrosis gene: Genetic analysis. *Science* **1989**, *245*, 1073–1080. [CrossRef]
11. Kloosterboer, M.; Hoffman, G.; Rock, M.; Gershan, W.; Laxova, A.; Li, Z.; Farrell, P.M. Clarification of laboratory and clinical variables that influence cystic fibrosis newborn screening with initial analysis of immunoreactive trypsinogen. *Pediatrics* **2009**, *123*, e338–e346. [CrossRef]
12. Gregg, R.G.; Wilfond, B.S.; Farrell, P.M.; Laxova, A.; Hassemer, D.; Mischler, E.H. Application of DNA analysis in a population-screening program for neonatal diagnosis of cystic fibrosis (CF): Comparison of screening protocols. *Am. J. Hum. Genet.* **1993**, *52*, 616–626.
13. Comeau, A.M.; Parad, R.B.; Dorkin, H.L.; Dovey, M.; Gerstle, R.; Haver, K.; Lapey, A.; O'Sullivan, B.P.; Waltz, D.A.; Zwerdling, R.G.; et al. Population-based newborn screening for genetic disorders when multiple mutation DNA testing is incorporated: A cystic fibrosis newborn screening model demonstrating increased sensitivity but more carrier detections. *Pediatrics* **2004**, *113*, 1573–1581. [CrossRef]

14. Sommerburg, O.; Hammermann, J.; Lindner, M.; Stahl, M.; Muckenthaler, M.; Kohlmueller, D.; Happich, M.; Kulozik, A.E.; Stopsack, M.; Gahr, M.; et al. Five years of experience with biochemical cystic fibrosis newborn screening based on IRT/PAP in Germany. *Pediatr. Pulmonol.* **2015**, *50*, 655–664. [CrossRef]

15. Accurso, F.J.; Sontag, M.K.; Wagener, J.S. Complications associated with symptomatic diagnosis in infants with cystic fibrosis. *J. Pediatr.* **2005**, *147*, S37–S41. [CrossRef]

16. Chatfield, S.; Owen, G.; Ryley, H.C.; Williams, J.; Alfaham, M.; Goodchild, M.C.; Weller, P. Neonatal screening for cystic fibrosis in Wales and the West Midlands: Clinical assessment after five years of screening. *Arch. Dis. Child.* **1991**, *66*, 29–33. [CrossRef]

17. Farrell, P.M.; Kosorok, M.R.; Laxova, A.; Shen, G.; Koscik, R.E.; Bruns, W.T.; Splaingard, M.; Mischler, E.H. Nutritional benefits of neonatal screening for cystic fibrosis. Wisconsin Cystic Fibrosis Neonatal Screening Study Group. *N. Engl. J. Med.* **1997**, *337*, 963–969. [CrossRef]

18. Balfour-Lynn, I.M. Newborn screening for cystic fibrosis: Evidence for benefit. *Arch. Dis. Child.* **2008**, *93*, 7–10. [CrossRef]

19. Farrell, P.M.; Kosorok, M.R.; Rock, M.J.; Laxova, A.; Zeng, L.; Lai, H.C.; Hoffman, G.; Laessig, R.H.; Splaingard, M.L. Early diagnosis of cystic fibrosis through neonatal screening prevents severe malnutrition and improves long-term growth. Wisconsin Cystic Fibrosis Neonatal Screening Study Group. *Pediatrics* **2001**, *107*, 1–13. [CrossRef]

20. Farrell, P.M.; Lai, H.J.; Li, Z.; Kosorok, M.R.; Laxova, A.; Green, C.G.; Collins, J.; Hoffman, G.; Laessig, R.; Rock, M.J.; et al. Evidence on improved outcomes with early diagnosis of cystic fibrosis through neonatal screening: Enough is enough! *J. Pediatr.* **2005**, *147*, S30–S36. [CrossRef]

21. Sanders, D.B.; Zhang, Z.; Farrell, P.M.; Lai, H.J.; Wisconsin, C.F.N.S.G. Early life growth patterns persist for 12 years and impact pulmonary outcomes in cystic fibrosis. *J. Cyst. Fibros.* **2018**, *17*, 528–535. [CrossRef]

22. Kosorok, M.R.; Jalaluddin, M.; Farrell, P.M.; Shen, G.; Colby, C.E.; Laxova, A.; Rock, M.J.; Splaingard, M. Comprehensive analysis of risk factors for acquisition of Pseudomonas aeruginosa in young children with cystic fibrosis. *Pediatr. Pulmonol.* **1998**, *26*, 81–88. [CrossRef]

23. Rosenfeld, M.; Emerson, J.; McNamara, S.; Thompson, V.; Ramsey, B.W.; Morgan, W.; Gibson, R.L.; Group, E.S. Risk factors for age at initial Pseudomonas acquisition in the cystic fibrosis epic observational cohort. *J. Cyst. Fibros.* **2012**, *11*, 446–453. [CrossRef]

24. Baussano, I.; Tardivo, I.; Bellezza-Fontana, R.; Forneris, M.P.; Lezo, A.; Anfossi, L.; Castello, M.; Aleksandar, V.; Bignamini, E. Neonatal screening for cystic fibrosis does not affect time to first infection with Pseudomonas aeruginosa. *Pediatrics* **2006**, *118*, 888–895. [CrossRef]

25. Tluczek, A.; Orland, K.M.; Cavanagh, L. Psychosocial consequences of false-positive newborn screens for cystic fibrosis. *Qual. Health Res.* **2011**, *21*, 174–186. [CrossRef]

26. Johnson, F.; Southern, K.W.; Ulph, F. Psychological impact on parents of an inconclusive diagnosis following newborn bloodspot screening for cystic fibrosis: A qualitative study. *Int. J. Neonatal Screen.* **2019**, *5*, 23. [CrossRef]

27. Tluczek, A.; Clark, R.; McKechnie, A.C.; Brown, R.L. Factors affecting parent-child relationships one year after positive newborn screening for cystic fibrosis or congenital hypothyroidism. *J. Dev. Behav. Pediatr.* **2015**, *36*, 24–34. [CrossRef]

28. Tluczek, A.; Laxova, A.; Grieve, A.; Heun, A.; Brown, R.L.; Rock, M.J.; Gershan, W.M.; Farrell, P.M. Long-term follow-up of cystic fibrosis newborn screening: Psychosocial functioning of adolescents and young adults. *J. Cyst. Fibros.* **2014**, *13*, 227–234. [CrossRef]

29. Ciske, D.J.; Haavisto, A.; Laxova, A.; Rock, L.Z.; Farrell, P.M. Genetic counseling and neonatal screening for cystic fibrosis: An assessment of the communication process. *Pediatrics* **2001**, *107*, 699–705. [CrossRef]

30. Munck, A.; Mayell, S.J.; Winters, V.; Shawcross, A.; Derichs, N.; Parad, R.; Barben, J.; Southern, K.W.; ECFS Neonatal Screening Working Group. Cystic Fibrosis Screen Positive, Inconclusive Diagnosis (CFSPID): A new designation and management recommendations for infants with an inconclusive diagnosis following newborn screening. *J. Cyst. Fibros.* **2015**, *14*, 706–713. [CrossRef]

31. Castellani, C.; Duff, A.J.A.; Bell, S.C.; Heijerman, H.G.M.; Munck, A.; Ratjen, F.; Sermet-Gaudelus, I.; Southern, K.W.; Barben, J.; Flume, P.A.; et al. ECFS best practice guidelines: The 2018 revision. *J. Cyst. Fibros.* **2018**, *17*, 153–178. [CrossRef]

32. David, J.; Chrastina, P.; Peskova, K.; Kozich, V.; Friedecky, D.; Adam, T.; Hlidkova, E.; Vinohradska, H.; Novotna, D.; Hedelova, M.; et al. Epidemiology of rare diseases detected by newborn screening in the Czech Republic. *Cent. Eur. J. Public Health* **2019**, *27*, 153–159. [CrossRef]
33. Scotet, V.; Dugueperoux, I.; Saliou, P.; Rault, G.; Roussey, M.; Audrezet, M.P.; Ferec, C. Evidence for decline in the incidence of cystic fibrosis: A 35-year observational study in Brittany, France. *Orphanet J. Rare Dis.* **2012**, *7*, 14. [CrossRef]
34. De Boeck, K. Cystic fibrosis in the year 2020: A disease with a new face. *Acta Paediatr.* **2020**. [CrossRef]
35. CLSI. *Newborn Screening for Cystic Fibrosis*, 2nd ed.; CLSI Guideline NBS05; CLSI: Wayne, PA, USA, 2019.
36. Ren, C.L.; Borowitz, D.S.; Gonska, T.; Howenstine, M.S.; Levy, H.; Massie, J.; Milla, C.; Munck, A.; Southern, K.W. Cystic Fibrosis Transmembrane Conductance Regulator-Related Metabolic Syndrome and Cystic Fibrosis Screen Positive, Inconclusive Diagnosis. *J. Pediatr.* **2017**, *181S*, S45–S51. [CrossRef]
37. Romeo, G.; Devoto, M.; Galietta, L.J. Why is the cystic fibrosis gene so frequent? *Hum. Genet.* **1989**, *84*, 1–5. [CrossRef]
38. Southern, K.W.; Munck, A.; Pollitt, R.; Travert, G.; Zanolla, L.; Dankert-Roelse, J.; Castellani, C.; ECFS CF Neonatal Screening Working Group. A survey of newborn screening for cystic fibrosis in Europe. *J. Cyst. Fibros.* **2007**, *6*, 57–65. [CrossRef]
39. Farrell, P.; Joffe, S.; Foley, L.; Canny, G.J.; Mayne, P.; Rosenberg, M. Diagnosis of cystic fibrosis in the Republic of Ireland: Epidemiology and costs. *Ir. Med. J.* **2007**, *100*, 557–560.
40. Newsletter ECFS Neonatal Screening Working Group. January 2014. Available online: https://www.ecfs.eu/sites/default/files/general-content-files/working-groups/NSWG_newsletter06Jan14.pdf (accessed on 1 March 2020).
41. Lucotte, G.; Hazout, S.; De Braekeleer, M. Complete map of cystic fibrosis mutation DF508 frequencies in Western Europe and correlation between mutation frequencies and incidence of disease. *Hum. Biol.* **1995**, *67*, 797–803.
42. Audrezet, M.P.; Munck, A.; Scotet, V.; Claustres, M.; Roussey, M.; Delmas, D.; Ferec, C.; Desgeorges, M. Comprehensive *CFTR* gene analysis of the French cystic fibrosis screened newborn cohort: Implications for diagnosis, genetic counseling, and mutation-specific therapy. *Genet. Med.* **2015**, *17*, 108–116. [CrossRef]
43. Castellani, C.; Picci, L.; Tridello, G.; Casati, E.; Tamanini, A.; Bartoloni, L.; Scarpa, M.; Assael, B.M.; Veneto, C.F.L.N. Cystic fibrosis carrier screening effects on birth prevalence and newborn screening. *Genet. Med.* **2016**, *18*, 145–151. [CrossRef]
44. Terlizzi, V.; Mergni, G.; Buzzetti, R.; Centrone, C.; Zavataro, L.; Braggion, C. Cystic fibrosis screen positive inconclusive diagnosis (CFSPID): Experience in Tuscany, Italy. *J. Cyst. Fibros.* **2019**, *18*, 484–490. [CrossRef]
45. Bauca, J.M.; Morell-Garcia, D.; Vila, M.; Perez, G.; Heine-Suner, D.; Figuerola, J. Assessing the improvements in the newborn screening strategy for cystic fibrosis in the Balearic Islands. *Clin. Biochem.* **2015**, *48*, 419–424. [CrossRef]
46. Skov, M.; Baekvad-Hansen, M.; Hougaard, D.M.; Skogstrand, K.; Lund, A.M.; Pressler, T.; Olesen, H.V.; Duno, M. Cystic fibrosis newborn screening in Denmark: Experience from the first 2 years. *Pediatr. Pulmonol.* **2020**, *55*, 549–555. [CrossRef]
47. Dankert-Roelse, J.E.; Bouva, M.J.; Jakobs, B.S.; Janssens, H.M.; de Winter-de Groot, K.M.; Schonbeck, Y.; Gille, J.J.P.; Gulmans, V.A.M.; Verschoof-Puite, R.K.; Schielen, P.; et al. Newborn blood spot screening for cystic fibrosis with a four-step screening strategy in the Netherlands. *J. Cyst. Fibros.* **2019**, *18*, 54–63. [CrossRef]
48. Sobczynska-Tomaszewska, A.; Oltarzewski, M.; Czerska, K.; Wertheim-Tysarowska, K.; Sands, D.; Walkowiak, J.; Bal, J.; Mazurczak, T.; NBS CF Working Group. Newborn screening for cystic fibrosis: Polish 4 years' experience with CFTR sequencing strategy. *Eur. J. Hum. Genet.* **2013**, *21*, 391–396. [CrossRef]
49. Soltysova, A.; Tothova Tarova, E.; Ficek, A.; Baldovic, M.; Polakova, H.; Kayserova, H.; Kadasi, L. Comprehensive genetic study of cystic fibrosis in Slovak patients in 25 years of genetic diagnostics. *Clin. Respir. J.* **2018**, *12*, 1197–1206. [CrossRef]
50. Lannefors, L.; Lindgren, A. Demographic transition of the Swedish cystic fibrosis community–results of modern care. *Respir. Med.* **2002**, *96*, 681–685. [CrossRef]
51. Marcao, A.; Barreto, C.; Pereira, L.; Guedes Vaz, L.; Cavaco, J.; Casimiro, A.; Felix, M.; Reis Silva, T.; Barbosa, T.; Freitas, C.; et al. Cystic fibrosis newborn screening in Portugal: PAP value in populations with stringent rules for genetic studies. *Int. J. Neonatal Screen.* **2018**, *4*, 22. [CrossRef]

52. Lundman, E.; Gaup, H.J.; Bakkeheim, E.; Olafsdottir, E.J.; Rootwelt, T.; Storrosten, O.T.; Pettersen, R.D. Implementation of newborn screening for cystic fibrosis in Norway. Results from the first three years. *J. Cyst. Fibros.* **2016**, *15*, 318–324. [CrossRef]
53. Popa, I.; Pop, L.; Popa, Z.; Schwarz, M.J.; Hambleton, G.; Malone, G.M.; Haworth, A.; Super, M. Cystic fibrosis mutations in Romania. *Eur. J. Pediatr.* **1997**, *156*, 212–213. [CrossRef]
54. Kere, J.; Estivill, X.; Chillon, M.; Morral, N.; Nunes, V.; Norio, R.; Savilahti, E.; de la Chapelle, A. Cystic fibrosis in a low-incidence population: Two major mutations in Finland. *Hum. Genet.* **1994**, *93*, 162–166. [CrossRef]
55. Barben, J.; Castellani, C.; Dankert-Roelse, J.; Gartner, S.; Kashirskaya, N.; Linnane, B.; Mayell, S.; Munck, A.; Sands, D.; Sommerburg, O.; et al. The expansion and performance of national newborn screening programmes for cystic fibrosis in Europe. *J. Cyst. Fibros.* **2017**, *16*, 207–213. [CrossRef]
56. Wilcken, B.; Wiley, V.; Sherry, G.; Bayliss, U. Neonatal screening for cystic fibrosis: A comparison of two strategies for case detection in 1.2 million babies. *J. Pediatr.* **1995**, *127*, 965–970. [CrossRef]
57. Massie, R.J.; Curnow, L.; Glazner, J.; Armstrong, D.S.; Francis, I. Lessons learned from 20 years of newborn screening for cystic fibrosis. *Med. J. Aust.* **2012**, *196*, 67–70. [CrossRef]
58. Wesley, A.W.; Stewart, A.W. Cystic fibrosis in New Zealand: Incidence and mortality. *N. Z. Med. J.* **1985**, *98*, 321–323.
59. Kosorok, M.R.; Wei, W.H.; Farrell, P.M. The incidence of cystic fibrosis. *Stat. Med.* **1996**, *15*, 449–462. [CrossRef]
60. Lilley, M.; Christian, S.; Hume, S.; Scott, P.; Montgomery, M.; Semple, L.; Zuberbuhler, P.; Tabak, J.; Bamforth, F.; Somerville, M.J. Newborn screening for cystic fibrosis in Alberta: Two years of experience. *Paediatr. Child Health* **2010**, *15*, 590–594. [CrossRef]
61. Eyheramendy, S.; Martinez, F.I.; Manevy, F.; Vial, C.; Repetto, G.M. Genetic structure characterization of Chileans reflects historical immigration patterns. *Nat. Commun.* **2015**, *6*, 6472. [CrossRef]
62. Lay-Son, G.; Puga, A.; Astudillo, P.; Repetto, G.M.; Collaborative Group of the Chilean National Cystic Fibrosis Program. Cystic fibrosis in Chilean patients: Analysis of 36 common CFTR gene mutations. *J. Cyst. Fibros.* **2011**, *10*, 66–70. [CrossRef]
63. Silva Filho, L.V.; Castanos, C.; Ruiz, H.H. Cystic fibrosis in Latin America-Improving the awareness. *J. Cyst. Fibros.* **2016**, *15*, 791–793. [CrossRef]
64. Nazer, H.M. Early diagnosis of cystic fibrosis in Jordanian children. *J. Trop. Pediatr.* **1992**, *38*, 113–115. [CrossRef]
65. Al-Mahroos, F. Cystic fibrosis in Bahrain incidence, phenotype, and outcome. *J. Trop. Pediatr.* **1998**, *44*, 35–39. [CrossRef]
66. Frossard, P.M.; Lestringant, G.; Girodon, E.; Goossens, M.; Dawson, K.P. Determination of the prevalence of cystic fibrosis in the United Arab Emirates by genetic carrier screening. *Clin. Genet.* **1999**, *55*, 496–497. [CrossRef]
67. Stafler, P.; Mei-Zahav, M.; Wilschanski, M.; Mussaffi, H.; Efrati, O.; Lavie, M.; Shoseyov, D.; Cohen-Cymberknoh, M.; Gur, M.; Bentur, L.; et al. The impact of a national population carrier screening program on cystic fibrosis birth rate and age at diagnosis: Implications for newborn screening. *J. Cyst. Fibros.* **2016**, *15*, 460–466. [CrossRef]
68. Goodchild, M.C.; Insley, J.; Rushton, D.I.; Gaze, H. Cystic fibrosis in 3 Pakistani children. *Arch. Dis. Child.* **1974**, *49*, 739–741. [CrossRef]
69. Powers, C.A.; Potter, E.M.; Wessel, H.U.; Lloyd-Still, J.D. Cystic fibrosis in Asian Indians. *Arch. Pediatr. Adolesc. Med.* **1996**, *150*, 554–555. [CrossRef]
70. Kapoor, V.; Shastri, S.S.; Kabra, M.; Kabra, S.K.; Ramachandran, V.; Arora, S.; Balakrishnan, P.; Deorari, A.K.; Paul, V.K. Carrier frequency of F508del mutation of cystic fibrosis in Indian population. *J. Cyst. Fibros.* **2006**, *5*, 43–46. [CrossRef]
71. Kabra, S.K.; Kabra, M.; Lodha, R.; Shastri, S. Cystic fibrosis in India. *Pediatr. Pulmonol.* **2007**, *42*, 1087–1094. [CrossRef]
72. Wright, S.W.; Morton, N.E. Genetic studies on cystic fibrosis in Hawaii. *Am. J. Hum. Genet.* **1968**, *20*, 157–169.
73. Yamashiro, Y.; Shimizu, T.; Oguchi, S.; Shioya, T.; Nagata, S.; Ohtsuka, Y. The estimated incidence of cystic fibrosis in Japan. *J. Pediatr. Gastroenterol. Nutr.* **1997**, *24*, 544–547. [CrossRef]

74. Liu, Y.; Wang, L.; Tian, X.; Xu, K.F.; Xu, W.; Li, X.; Yue, C.; Zhang, P.; Xiao, Y.; Zhang, X. Characterization of gene mutations and phenotypes of cystic fibrosis in Chinese patients. *Respirology* **2015**, *20*, 312–318. [CrossRef]
75. Singh, M.; Rebordosa, C.; Bernholz, J.; Sharma, N. Epidemiology and genetics of cystic fibrosis in Asia: In preparation for the next-generation treatments. *Respirology* **2015**, *20*, 1172–1181. [CrossRef]
76. Al-Sadeq, D.; Abunada, T.; Dalloul, R.; Fahad, S.; Taleb, S.; Aljassim, K.; Al Hamed, F.A.; Zayed, H. Spectrum of mutations of cystic fibrosis in the 22 Arab countries: A systematic review. *Respirology* **2019**, *24*, 127–136. [CrossRef]

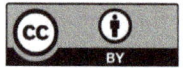

© 2020 by the authors. Licensee MDPI, Basel, Switzerland. This article is an open access article distributed under the terms and conditions of the Creative Commons Attribution (CC BY) license (http://creativecommons.org/licenses/by/4.0/).

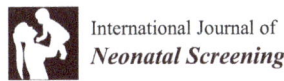

Review

Constructing a Bioethical Framework to Evaluate and Optimise Newborn Bloodspot Screening for Cystic Fibrosis

Rachael E. Armstrong [1], Lucy Frith [2], Fiona M. Ulph [3] and Kevin W. Southern [1,*]

1. Department of Women's and Children's Health, University of Liverpool, Liverpool L12 2AP, UK; r.armstrong3@doctors.org.uk
2. Institute of Population Health, University of Liverpool, Liverpool L69 3GL, UK; frith@liverpool.ac.uk
3. Division of Psychology & Mental Health, School of Health Sciences, Faculty of Biology, Medicine and Health, University of Manchester, Manchester Academic Health Science Centre, Manchester M13 9PL, UK; Fiona.Ulph@manchester.ac.uk
* Correspondence: kwsouth@liv.ac.uk; Tel.: +44-151-2933536

Received: 13 March 2020; Accepted: 4 May 2020; Published: 26 May 2020

Abstract: Newborn bloodspot screening for cystic fibrosis is a valid public health strategy for populations with a high incidence of this inherited condition. There are a wide variety of approaches to screening and in this paper, we propose that a bioethical framework is required to determine the most appropriate screening protocol for a population. This framework depends on the detailed evaluation of the ethical consequences of all screening outcomes and placing these in the context of the genetic profile of the population screened, the geography of the region and the healthcare resources available.

Keywords: cystic fibrosis; newborn bloodspot screening; cystic fibrosis screen positive; inconclusive diagnosis (CFSPID); bioethics

1. Introduction

In this paper, we develop a bioethical framework that can be used to assess newborn bloodspot screening (NBS) for cystic fibrosis (CF) protocols [1,2]. This approach provides a means to appraise the impact of the evolving technologies that are increasingly being used as part of screening protocols, for example more extensive DNA analyses [3]. An ethical consideration is essential for all screening strategies but particularly pertinent for NBS for CF for three main reasons: (1) NBS for CF protocols are complex and varied, (2) expanded DNA analysis including sequencing is increasingly common and (3) outcomes are complicated and not comprehensively recognised or characterised.

The measurement of immuno-reactive trypsinogen (IRT) from a dried bloodspot (DBS) sample enabled screening for CF by providing a simple and inexpensive test, as per the criteria outlined by the World Health Organisation (WHO) [4]. However, other criteria outlined by Wilson and Jungner were more challenging to fulfil, namely that an early diagnosis following a positive NBS resulted in improved outcomes for children with CF. This felt at odds with the lived experience of regions in which NBS for CF was established, when qualitatively the impact of an earlier diagnosis seemed considerable [5].

In an important study undertaken in Wisconsin (USA), over 650,000 DBS samples were analysed for IRT (and in some cases DNA analysis), but only results from alternative samples were reported [6]. In 54 of the samples reported, a positive NBS result was associated with an early diagnosis and significantly improved nutritional outcomes, compared to 67 infants diagnosed clinically. These early differences in nutritional well-being were transient, reflecting the capacity of standard care to address the early challenges of growth delay in clinically diagnosed children [7]. There were no clinically significant differences in respiratory outcomes, and this was consistent with a study undertaken in the United Kingdom [8,9].

For those who work in the field, there was a disconnection between the apparent positive impact of NBS in the clinical environment and the relative lack of evidence for improved outcomes for people with CF after NBS. To some degree, this reflects the ability of CF teams and parents to provide high quality CF care following a clinical diagnosis, even if delayed [9]. However, evidence is increasing that small differences in clinical outcomes in the early months of life can lead to significant and sometimes dramatic differences in outcomes later in life. This is supported by the historical cohort study undertaken in Australia that compared two groups of children with CF before and after the implementation of NBS for CF [10]. Over the first two decades, differences between the two cohorts were minimal, but a distinct and large difference in survival became apparent as the cohorts entered their adult years, with the clinically diagnosed group faring much less well. These data are supported by data from other programmes, including an Italian group reinforcing the view that early recognition and treatment through NBS may have a more profound impact on clinical outcomes later in life [11,12] (Figure 1).

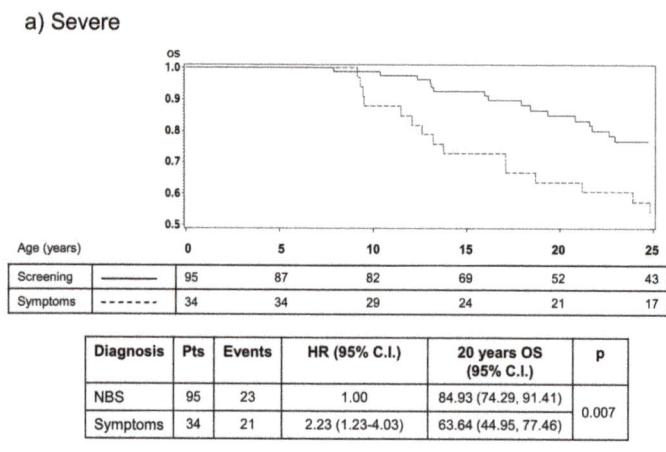

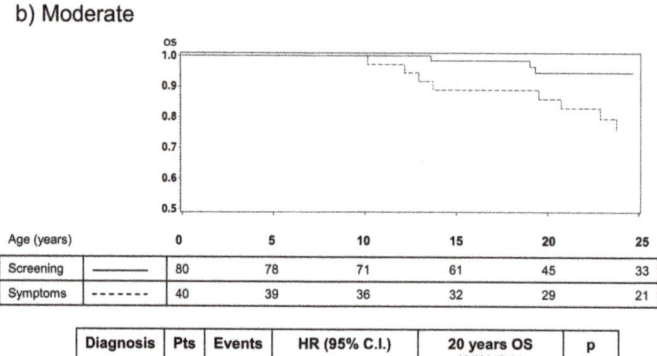

Figure 1. *Cont.*

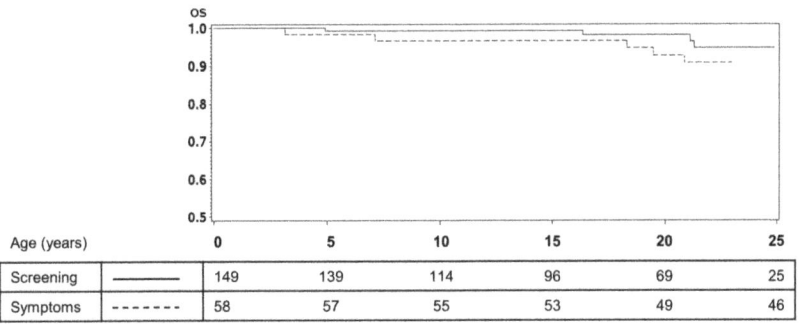

Figure 1. Results from an Italian study that illustrates the impact of early diagnosis through NBS on survival. The impact on survival is most apparent in infants with severe (**a**) or moderate disease (**b**) after diagnosis, highlighting the reduced impact of early diagnosis on people with mild or less typical CF (**c**) [12].

There are other important but "softer" outcomes that support the rationale of NBS for CF—namely, preventing the diagnostic odyssey that many families have to endure, providing families with information to inform future reproductive decisions and providing a framework for improved and more systematic CF services to be established across a region [1].

On the basis of these data, there is a compelling rationale to support NBS for CF, but also a responsibility to ensure that protocols are designed to minimise negative outcomes [1]. It is clear that the WHO screening criteria alone are not sufficient to critically judge the validity of a programme. Petros suggests an expanded list of criteria which provides a more comprehensive picture of the worth of an NBS programme [13]. Using these criteria, he argues that NBS for CF is a valid and worthwhile undertaking. These additional criteria are helpful, but still not adequate to rigorously evaluate a programme in the era of new emerging technologies, especially the ability to undertake extensive DNA testing in a cheap and timely manner. Advances in the capability to undertake extensive genetic testing have outpaced the capacity of most to assimilate this knowledge, and for many it is a potential cause of significant anxiety [14]. In such a climate, we propose that a bioethical approach is required to provide a framework to assess and optimise NBS for CF to ensure that the most appropriate protocol is used for a given population.

To work towards a bioethical framework, it is important to consider the impact of all possible outcomes from NBS for CF both in isolation and collectively, weighing up the relative importance to society and individuals. To establish a framework, we examined all potential outcomes for NBS for CF and related these to ethical considerations.

This work was undertaken in a series of small group meetings between the author team, with subsequent email correspondence and a literature review.

2. Outcomes from Newborn Bloodspot Screening for CF

Below, we list the potential outcomes from NBS for CF and the bioethical issues raised by each.

2.1. True Negative: An Infant with a Negative NBS Result, Not Affected by CF

An effective outcome of the screening programme is the accurate exclusion of cystic fibrosis. The accurate identification of infants who do not have CF is a positive outcome with no associated adverse consequences. As with all screening, this societal benefit is accepted and often underappreciated by the general population.

2.2. True Positive: An Infant with CF Detected by NBS

Early diagnosis provides a window of opportunity for proactive nutritional intervention. The impact on well-being later in life is now becoming apparent, as outlined in the introduction.

The beneficial implications of a true positive NBS result are:

- Proactive treatment.
- An earlier diagnostic period provides an opportunity to initiate an earlier referral into specialist tertiary care centres and to start positive intervention at the earliest opportunity.
- Preventing a potentially protracted and painful diagnostic journey.
- Diagnostic delays for children affected by cystic fibrosis have been shown to be associated with negative psychosocial consequences [15]. The journey to a clinical diagnosis may be protracted and more complicated, with higher levels of psychological distress for the individual and family. The early detection of CF in a newborn prevents this by providing a timely diagnosis and access to the appropriate specialist CF team [16].
- Information for reproductive decision making.
- A positive NBS result, subsequently confirmed by diagnostic assessment, provides an opportunity for the parents (and other family members) to obtain further information about the implications of CF and to have the option to consider future reproductive decisions. The parents should be provided with genetic counselling to guide them through this process, mitigate unaddressed fears and uncertainty and enable them to make informed decisions.

A potential negative impact of a true positive NBS result is the possibility of revealing non-paternity (for example, an infant is recognised to be homozygous for F508del, but subsequent genetic testing of the parents demonstrates that the father is not a carrier). Although this is a rare negative compared to the considerable positive impact, it is important that appropriate follow up is in place for parents to seek genetic counselling and support following the NBS process, and this should be empathetic and sensitive.

Whilst a true positive result is of benefit to the infant and family, this needs to be balanced with the potential for harm. Parents/carers may consider that they have had time with a "normal" child diminished, and the initial processing of a positive result needs to be handled sensitively, with a particular focus on timeliness and clear information. It is important that this situation is not presented to families as a "good news story" that their child has been diagnosed early, and neither should it be presented dramatically. Rather, it should be presented as the start of a journey to a hopefully full and active life. The communication of the result and the subsequent diagnostic assessment is a task requiring experience and skill, and some parents are particularly vulnerable at this point. Healthcare professionals should be able to recognise this and address the parents' needs appropriately over time.

It is essential that a newly diagnosed infant with CF has access to high quality CF care which does not place them at risk (for example, from cross infection with airway pathogens). Health economic analysis demonstrates that whilst infants with CF recognised through NBS may have similar outcomes to those diagnosed clinically, this is at the expense of less treatment intervention (i.e., clinically diagnosed infants need more treatment to achieve similar outcomes) [17]. Hence, a societal benefit is achieved. It is clear that from a bioethical view, a true positive result achieves considerable individual and societal benefit but occasional harm; programmes must strive to minimise harm (non-maleficence).

2.3. Recognition of an Infant as a Carrier (Negative NBS Result)

For some programmes (for example, The Netherlands and UK), carrier reporting is a possible outcome. For most programmes using DNA analysis as a second tier of testing, carriers are only confirmed after clinical assessment and sweat testing. For these families, this result would be consistent with a false positive experience (see next section). Carrier reporting may leave the family with some anxiety around the possibility of an unrecognised second Cystic Fibrosis Transmembrane Conductance Regulator (CFTR) variant, and clear information is required to minimise this potential harm.

The detection of carrier status in a baby provides an opportunity for the parents to undergo genetic counselling and testing, which may impact on future reproductive decision making and cascade screening for other family members. There is a potential for negative impact arising from carrier recognition. There is evidence of increased parental anxiety about the child; in one study, a significant number of parents (18%) felt anxious about the health of their child four years after screening, suggesting a lack of assimilation of the "healthy carrier" concept [18]. The delivery and communication of carrier status are key factors, with most concern being caused by uncertainty or confusion regarding the use of negative terms such as "query" around the screening result [19]. A perceived negative style of communication from the healthcare professional can cause increased anxiety, and lead to family issues (stigma), depression and relationship difficulties [20]. Indeed, this study suggested that parents do not perceive the information that their child is a carrier as negative, rather, the distress arises from communication practices. Concerns for the family include anxiety about the status of their other children and how to communicate the result with other family members [21]. This work found that whilst some families could be very supportive, other families could find this communication very challenging and may effectively "shut down" conversations, blame the person starting the conversation, or increase existing family stress. Providing effective support for people could lead to families benefiting from the information rather than it becoming a disruptive factor.

As with a true positive result, carrier recognition is associated with the potential risk of recognising non-paternity. This needs to be considered in the processing of a carrier result, for example leaving further genetic counselling as an option to the parents rather than making it compulsory, as in some programmes.

An ethical issue raised by all newborn screening is the possibility of reducing autonomy, as those screened have no opportunity for consent or control over the data generated. Self-determination does not feature in these public health screening strategies. This is balanced against the rights of children to receive optimal healthcare. Carrier recognition throws this into sharp relief, and the ownership of this information requires careful consideration. It is imperative that young adults identified as carriers through NBS receive this information in a clear and sensitive manner. At present, there is no clear guidance for programmes on this issue on what information and in what format to pass on [22]. It is assumed to be the responsibility of the adults who receive the initial result (parent/carers and primary healthcare professionals), who may not appreciate or want to pass on the information. As there is no clear guidance on how to manage this situation, there is a potential for harm when the index case becomes aware of their carrier status or if they are denied information on which to make fully informed decisions about their reproductive options.

2.4. False Positive: An Infant with a Positive NBS Result, Who Does Not Have CF

False positive NBS results are associated with acute psychological distress for the parent/carers, and for some this may extend into longer-term psychological morbidity [23]. The period of time between a false positive NBS result and the subsequent diagnostic testing has been shown to be acutely stressful for the family [24]. Qualitative research has shown that parents experience feelings of guilt for having passed on a "faulty" gene, and that even following confirmative diagnostic testing to exclude

CF, they still harbour feelings of scepticism and fear that the test may be wrong, with subsequent anxiety for their child's health. This may affect how parents perceive and respond to healthcare services in the future, and may undermine their confidence in medical services [23,25].

A population-based cohort study reported higher maternal worry scores for mothers with an infant with a false positive NBS result and, even following adjustment for confounding variables, there was a higher proportion of parents using outpatient and accident and emergency services for infants with a false positive NBS result compared to matched controls [26]. Care should be taken to ensure parents are fully informed in the antenatal period about the screening process and subsequent diagnostic testing, in order to avoid misconceptions about the screening result and prevent psychosocial confusion and the over-medicalisation of healthy infants [19]. In one prospective study, 96% of parents expressed having been anxious at the time of being informed about the need for a diagnostic sweat test, and the anxiety increased proportionally to the waiting time for diagnostic testing; 86% felt entirely reassured three months after the test. This suggests that the distress associated with a false positive result is most likely to be temporary [27]. Participants in a qualitative study have commented that they would be willing to endure the acute psychosocial risks of a false positive result in acknowledgement of the potential value of a true positive result and the recognition of the health benefits of an early diagnosis [23,26].

Families who remained anxious 3 months after diagnostic testing described doubts regarding the test's reliability, a poor understanding of the screening and diagnostic process and fears of CF being transmitted to future generations [27]. To minimise undermining parental confidence in the healthcare system, it is important to counsel families about the screening process, particularly when the initial result requires further diagnostic confirmation; this is particularly important when the initial screening result is positive, as there is an increased potential for misconceptions and doubt about the reliability of further testing. This information and support needs to be provided antenatally and be reinforced throughout the pregnancy, birth and postnatal period.

A small subset of parents continued to have persisting concerns about the health implications for their child following a false positive NBS result; namely, concerns of the possibility of poor health and illness for the infant, the fear of CF affecting another child or a genetic mutation affecting another family member, with some cases leading to a 'finger pointing' culture of attempting to identify the source of a suspected mutation [23]. It is important that screening programmes incorporate a recognition of the importance of counselling families on the meaning of a false positive NBS result, and that parents have the opportunity to express and discuss their concerns, with access to appropriate genetic counselling services where required.

Although, in general, the distress associated with a false positive result is considered transient, it may be that there are subtle longer-term psychosocial issues that quantitative studies may not have been sensitive enough to identify. Regardless, there is good agreement that NBS for all conditions should aim to minimise false positives. The European CF Society (ECFS) standards of care document suggests that CF programmes should aim for a positive predictive value greater than 0.3 (i.e., for every 10 infants with a positive NBS result, more than three will have a confirmed diagnosis of CF) [28].

2.5. Unresolved Cases

In some cases, a positive NBS result may remain unresolved. For example, an extremely preterm infant may have a positive NBS result, with a raised IRT level and one CF-causing gene variant detected. The infant may die from complications of preterm birth before further diagnostic testing is possible. Although this is a rare event in screening programmes, the increased incidence of raised IRT measurements in sick infants and infants with profound chromosomal abnormalities makes this a situation that occurs more frequently than might be anticipated by chance [29].

An unresolved screening outcome may cause psychological morbidity for the affected parents. The significance of the screening result is unknown, potentially causing increased concerns for future reproductive decisions. In addition, this result is presented during a period of extreme distress for parents, who may be unable to assimilate the information correctly.

Unresolved anxieties and a lack of diagnostic certainty may contribute to longer-term psychological distress, particularly in the context of further reproductive decisions in the face of uncertain genetic information.

2.6. Cystic Fibrosis Screen Positive, Inconclusive Diagnosis (CFSPID)

A potential outcome from a positive NBS result is an inconclusive diagnosis [30,31]. The number of infants with an unclear diagnosis is dependent on the NBS approach taken, with increased recognition associated with increased DNA analysis [32]. For example, a protocol that employs extended gene sequencing will recognise more infants with an unclear diagnosis, and these infants will be more likely to remain well. Biochemical protocols with no DNA analysis will still recognise infants with an unclear diagnosis but at a much lower rate and with intermediate sweat test results (a sweat chloride concentration of between 30 and 59 mmol/L). Infants with an intermediate sweat chloride are more likely to develop clinical features consistent with CF and convert to a CF diagnosis [33].

A number of papers have considered the evaluation and management of these infants and this is covered in another chapter in this series, as are the issues around designation [34]. Recently, a global exercise resulted in the harmonisation of the definition and designation of these infants as Cystic Fibrosis Transmembrane Conductance Regulator (CFTR)-Related Metabolic Syndrome/Cystic Fibrosis Screen Positive, Inconclusive Diagnosis (CRMS/CFSPID) [30,31]. For this paper, we will use the term CFSPID.

Infants with a CFSPID designation are by definition healthy, and the majority will remain healthy through their childhood. There are three pathways that can lead to a conversion to a CF diagnosis:

1. A repeat sweat test becomes supportive of a CF diagnosis (sweat chloride >59 mmol/L).
2. New information emerges that the CFTR variant is CF-causing (two CF-causing variants equates to a CF diagnosis, regardless of the sweat chloride value).
3. The CFSPID infant develops symptoms consistent with a CF diagnosis (most commonly a chronic cough).

For a programme using extended gene sequencing, around 5% of the infants designated as CFSPID will convert to a CF diagnosis [25]. For programmes with limited or no DNA analysis, conversion is more common (between 25% and 40%), although total numbers will be less [33]. If a programme that employs extended gene sequencing only reports variants that are CF-causing, this will significantly reduce the recognition of infants with CFSPID.

The majority of infants who do not convert to a CF diagnosis face an increased risk of a CFTR-related disorder (CFTR-RD) later in their life. A CFTR-RD is defined as a condition (usually single organ) that is associated with abnormal CFTR function [35]. The most common example is the congenital bilateral absence of the vas deferens (CBAVD), which is a cause of male infertility. Other potential CFTR-RDs include pancreatitis and rhinosinusitis. The risk of developing these conditions is not currently quantifiable, and counselling families and CFSPID individuals about the long-term risk is challenging. Whilst possibly the information may represent some benefit to the family of an early diagnosis in some cases, overall the situation raises a number of ethical issues, not least those around autonomy and non-maleficence, with the risk of over-medicalisation and iatrogenic harm. Qualitative studies of parents in this situation have demonstrated the profound negative impact this designation has on health beliefs and behaviours and the undermining of trust in health professionals [36].

There is no evidence that recognition of CFSPID improves outcomes, although some argue that it empowers families to make health decisions. In light of this, the European Neonatal Screening Working Group suggested in their best practice document that NBS protocols should aim to minimise the recognition of CFSPID infants [37]. This may be achieved by only reporting CF-causing variants in larger DNA panels and not reporting carriers or variants of varying clinical consequence. This raises the issue of autonomy in not reporting a result, even if that result is unclear and screened out by a computer (algorithm independent of human awareness). There may be an ethical argument that such selective reporting improves the performance of the programme in other regards, for example positive predictive value (PPV) and therefore this is compensated by the reduction in false positives. Consensus documents provide evidence-based guidance on the management of CFSPID with advice that minimises the medicalisation of these families [34]. Despite this, CFSPID infants are at risk of iatrogenic harm through inappropriate investigation and treatment, counter to the ethical principle of non-maleficence.

It is too early to evaluate the impact of a CFSPID designation on the child as they grow, but there is certainly a risk of psychological morbidity if it is not handled sensitively. This will need research to characterise the impact and provide guidance.

2.7. False Negative: An Affected, Undetected Infant—An infant with CF Not Detected by NBS

The outcome of newborn screening with the most potential for harm is a false negative result. The number of affected but not detected infants is a key performance measure of a screening programme. For most programmes, the commonest cause of a false negative result is an initial IRT result that is below the cut-off for further testing [32]. This is dependent on the cut-off used and the age of the baby when the dried blood sample is taken (IRT levels fall over the first weeks of life). Decreasing the IRT cut-off may improve the sensitivity, but this will be at the expense of a potential reduction in specificity [32]. A balance needs to be achieved between the improved sensitivity from lowering the cut-off and the reduction in the positive predictive value. Deciding this requires the weighing of different ethical values. Other strategies can be utilised to improve PPV and these include more extended DNA analysis, but again this can impact on the performance of other aspects of the NBS. For example, in a region with an ethnically diverse population, unusual CFTR variants may be missed and the sensitivity reduced. An approach to counter this has been the use of a "safety net", where extremely high IRT values result in further diagnostic testing even if no CFTR mutations are recognized [1]. Whilst this strategy is employed by many programmes, again it can result in a reduction in PPV. It can be seen, therefore, that different approaches can have positive and negative impacts on sensitivity and these need to be carefully considered in the bioethical framework.

The potential negative impacts of a false negative NBS result:

- The infant may have nutritional compromise or an airway infection that may have been avoided with early recognition.
- In a region with established NBS for CF, physicians may be less likely to consider a CF diagnosis and the family may have a prolonged diagnostic journey.
- Non-Caucasian populations may be disadvantaged by the use of DNA panels designed for populations from a North European background [1].
- Parents are denied knowledge (that their child has CF) that may inform future reproductive decision making.
- A false negative result may undermine confidence in the healthcare service.

Programmes should establish robust mechanisms to collect false negative data in order to usefully evaluate the impact on the population. However, it is important that false negative results are considered in the context of other aspects of the programme and not over emphasised at the expense of other performance metrics.

3. The Importance of Clear Communication

Research has shown the importance of effective and open communication with relatives during the newborn screening process; for example, the reasons for persisting anxieties experienced by parents affected by a false positive result were given as uncertainty about the reliability of tests and a poor understanding of the screening and diagnostic process, showing the importance of clear and accurate communication. A study on false positive results showed that there was almost a universal perception of the newborn screening test as an "indispensable tool"; admittedly, this is for parents affected by a false positive result and therefore cannot be generalised to those affected by a false negative result, but this finding does demonstrate the importance of educating and informing relatives about the screening process [27]. Certainly, consensus guidelines highlight the importance of ensuring positive and effective communication with families, and this is seen as an imperative component of all newborn screening programmes for CF.

4. Achieving an Ethical Balance

There are elements of the NBS protocol that will impact on the performance of the screening programme (Table 1). These need to be considered when developing a programme in light of four main factors:

1. What is the geographical spread of the population?
2. What healthcare provision is accessible for the population?
3. What is the CFTR genetic profile of the population?
4. What is the capacity of a health system to provide clear information to parents/carers (antenatally, postnatally) and for the child as they grow into adult life?

Table 1. Factors to consider when designing a protocol for cystic fibrosis (CF) newborn bloodspot screening (NBS).

Factors that will improve the sensitivity of a CF NBS programme
• A lower threshold for the first IRT value
• An extensive DNA panel targeted for the population screened
• A safety net, when a very high IRT-1 sample triggers further testing even if second tier testing (DNA or pancreatitis-associated-protein (PAP)) is negative
Factors that will improve the positive predictive value of a CF NBS programme
• A higher IRT-1 threshold
• Obtaining the first DBS sample later
• A second IRT measurement (at day 14-21)
• Extended gene sequencing
• A second biochemical test like PAP
• Not screening pre-term infants
• Not using a safety net
Factors that will reduce carrier recognition
• A higher IRT-1 threshold (and a later DBS sample)
• No DNA analysis
• Reduced DNA panel as a first line
• A second IRT sample (day 14-21)
• An algorithm with extended sequencing where carriers are not reported
Factors that will reduce CFSPID recognition
• A higher IRT-1 threshold (and later sampling)
• A second biochemical test (PAP)
• Reduced DNA analysis
• Limiting reporting to CF causing variants after extended gene sequencing
• A second IRT sample (day 14-21)

The first question to address is: is it ethically justified to screen this population for CF? The incidence of CF in a population correlates well with the prevalence of the F508del variant. In populations with a low F508del prevalence, the incidence of CF will be low, and the ethical balance will be tilted towards not screening, as screening will result in more negative impacts (for example, a poor PPV) than positive (actual cases of CF identified). An example to consider is screening in populations from sub-Saharan Africa. Studies in the US have demonstrated higher IRT levels in black infants compared to other ethnic populations, and it is reasonable to translate those data to the majority of infants born in sub-Saharan Africa [38]. This population also has a low F508del prevalence, consistent with a low overall prevalence of CF. Screening newborns from this population will result in a disproportionate number of false positive results (poor PPV) and an increased CFSPID recognition, especially if a DNA-based protocol is used. Our ethical framework clearly does not support NBS for CF in this population at present, as the balance of limited benefit is outweighed by the significant negative impact of diagnostic uncertainty and false positive tests for many families.

The decision to screen or not to screen is also influenced by the factors above; for example, if the family are geographically accessible and the healthcare infrastructure means the family can be visited to obtain a second DBS, then it may be possible to design a programme with improved PPV that is ethically acceptable. The "standards of care" published by the ECFS suggest that with an incidence of above 1 in 7000 births, the appropriateness of NBS for CF should be considered [28].

The geographical location and the framework of healthcare provision both impact on the capability to undertake a second DBS and high-quality sweat testing. These are important considerations when determining the ethical balance of a programme (Table 1). For example, if the programme is screening a geographically dispersed population with limited access to diagnostic testing, a protocol with good PPV, ideally from a single DBS sample, would be preferred from an ethical perspective, even at the expense of reduced sensitivity. In Turkey, because of the low F508del prevalence in the population, it was decided to implement a two stage IRT-IRT protocol. In most areas of the country, this required the family to travel to a local health centre for the collection of the second DBS sample, as it was not universally possible for a healthcare professional to travel to the family home. This subsequently resulted in a number of families not attending and incomplete testing. Establishing an IRT-IRT protocol reduced some of the harms associated with the recognition of CFSPID, but the inability to complete the protocol in some cases, together with a low PPV, raises an ethical discussion to consider the balance of this approach [39].

It is important that a country has an adequate health infra-structure to provide a good standard of care for infants with a positive NBS result and diagnosis of CF, although there should be a recognition that, in some countries, the implementation of NBS for CF may result in the development of better services to care for children with CF. The NBS process facilitates the regional concentration of positive results and improved utilisation of resources. Finally, it is important that NBS for CF is sensitive to the cultural and religious composition of a region.

5. Discussion

Newborn bloodspot screening for CF is complex, and there are numerous options for the screening protocol design. Surveys by the ECFS Neonatal Screening Working Group have identified over 50 different protocols in Europe [32]. It is clear that NBS for CF fulfils the traditional and more recent criteria that are used to determine the appropriateness of screening [13]. However, in this paper we have outlined the need for a bioethical consideration of this public health intervention to better determine the most appropriate protocol for a given population. Protocols should be assessed by considering the balance between beneficence (achieving a positive impact), non-maleficence (restricting the negative impacts) and the justice and autonomy of the parents, child and wider family. It is important to characterise and acknowledge the negative outcomes recorded in this paper in order to design the most appropriate programme for a population.

To design an ethical framework for screening is a multifaceted conceptual process, one which requires consideration of the impact of an intervention on the individual, family and society, and with perspectives that encompass the biological, psychological and social facets of the intervention. The consideration of beneficence and non-maleficence must be balanced against societal justice and the rights of the individual to benefit from early recognition and treatment of their condition, as well as self-determination.

This framework begins by addressing the ethical implications of each screening outcome, as outlined in the body of this article. This provides a guideline for those involved in the design or evaluation of newborn screening for CF and outlines the implications that ought to be considered and evaluated. The next step is to consider how to weigh the different outcomes and what ethical values should guide this, how to determine which factors should be given more significance, and how this impacts the overall outcome of the evaluation. Achieving this practice requires wide stakeholder engagement and discussion. This will allow a flexible, reflective evaluation that can be applied to programmes designed for varying populations. Once the relative ethical acceptability of the different outcomes has been determined, the next phase of the project will be using the framework to evaluate the active current screening programmes in order to determine the validity and effectiveness of the proposed framework. It is important that programmes critically review performance and adjust accordingly if they are not achieving the anticipated outcomes. Many programmes are resistant to change, but there are good examples of programmes that have adjusted cut-offs and DNA panels in light of sub-optimal performances. The national programme in France is an excellent example of a well performing programme that improved its "ethical balance" through a critical appraisal of its performance [40].

6. Conclusions

The complexities of newborn screening need to be considered and discussed in order to ensure the process of screening is ethical, fair, acceptable and just. The variety of potential approaches to screening introduces further complexity, and the ethical acceptability of the different outcomes will differ depending on the population screened. It is important to evaluate the process of NBS for CF and pay particular attention to the unintended consequences, including false negative results, carrier recognition and unresolved or inconclusive cases. We propose a framework for ethically evaluating NBS programmes that considers all the possible outcomes and evaluates their significance. The next step requires determining the relative acceptability of these outcomes, which will vary depending on the population; these can only be established for each population through stakeholder engagement. The framework can then be used to guide the design and evaluation of screening programmes. This framework will help guide policymakers to determine the most ethically acceptable programme, and to help identify, acknowledge and ameliorate the consequences of each outcome.

Funding: This research received no funding.

Conflicts of Interest: The authors declare no conflict of interest.

References

1. Castellani, C.; Massie, J.; Sontag, M.; Southern, K.W. Newborn screening for cystic fibrosis. *Lancet Respir. Med.* **2016**, *4*, 653–661. [CrossRef]
2. Goldenberg, A.J.; Lloyd-Puryear, M.; Brosco, J.P.; Therrell, B.; Bush, L.; Berry, S.; Brower, A.; Bonhomme, N.; Bowdish, B.; Clarke, A.; et al. Including ELSI research questions in newborn screening pilot studies. *Genet. Med.* **2019**, *21*, 525–533. [CrossRef]
3. Bell, S.C.; Mall, M.A.; Gutierrez, H.; Macek, M.; Madge, S.; Davies, J.C.; Burgel, P.R.; Tullis, E.; Castaños, C.; Byrnes, C.A.; et al. The future of cystic fibrosis care: A global perspective. *Lancet Respir. Med.* **2020**, *8*, 65–124. [CrossRef]
4. Wilson, J.M.; Jungner, Y.G. Principles and practice of mass screening for disease. *Bol Oficina Sanit Panam* **1968**, *65*, 281–393. [PubMed]
5. Hammond, K.B.; Abman, S.H.; Sokol, R.J.; Accurso, F.J. Efficacy of statewide neonatal screening for cystic fibrosis by assay of trypsinogen concentrations. *N. Engl. J. Med.* **1991**, *325*, 769–774. [CrossRef] [PubMed]

6. Farrell, P.M.; Kosorok, M.R.; Laxova, A.; Shen, G.; Koscik, R.E.; Bruns, W.T.; Splaingard, M.; Mischler, E.H.; Wisconsin Cystic Fibrosis Neonatal Screening Study Group. Nutritional benefits of neonatal screening for cystic fibrosis. *N. Engl. J. Med.* **1997**, *337*, 963–969. [CrossRef] [PubMed]
7. Farrell, P.M.; Kosorok, M.R.; Rock, M.J.; Laxova, A.; Zeng, L.; Lai, H.C.; Hoffman, G.; Laessig, R.H.; Splaingard, M.L.; Wisconsin Cystic Fibrosis Neonatal Screening Study Group. Early diagnosis of cystic fibrosis through neonatal screening prevents severe malnutrition and improves long-term growth. *Pediatrics* **2001**, *107*, 1–13. [CrossRef]
8. Farrell, P.M.; Li, Z.; Kosorok, M.R.; Laxova, A.; Green, C.G.; Collins, J.; Lai, H.-C.; Rock, M.J.; Splaingard, M.L. Bronchopulmonary disease in children with cystic fibrosis after early or delayed diagnosis. *Am. J. Respir. Crit. Care Med.* **2003**, *168*, 1100–1108. [CrossRef] [PubMed]
9. Chatfield, S.; Owen, G.; Ryley, H.C.; Williams, J.; Alfaham, M.; Goodchild, M.C.; Weller, P. Neonatal screening for cystic fibrosis in Wales and the West Midlands: Clinical assessment after five years of screening. *Arch. Dis. Child.* **1991**, *66*, 29–33. [CrossRef]
10. Dijk, F.N.; McKay, K.; Barzi, F.; Gaskin, K.J.; Fitzgerald, D.A. Improved survival in cystic fibrosis patients diagnosed by newborn screening compared to a historical cohort from the same centre. *Arch. Dis. Child.* **2011**, *96*, 1118–1123. [CrossRef]
11. Sanders, D.B.; Zhang, Z.; Farrell, P.M.; Lai, H.J.; Wisconsin, C.F.N.S.G. Early life growth patterns persist for 12 years and impact pulmonary outcomes in cystic fibrosis. *J. Cyst. Fibros.* **2018**, *17*, 528–535. [CrossRef] [PubMed]
12. Tridello, G.; Castellani, C.; Meneghelli, I.; Tamanini, A.; Assael, B.M. Early diagnosis from newborn screening maximises survival in severe cystic fibrosis. *ERJ Open Res.* **2018**, *4*. [CrossRef] [PubMed]
13. Petros, M. Revisiting the Wilson-Jungner criteria: How can supplemental criteria guide public health in the era of genetic screening? *Genet. Med.* **2012**, *14*, 129–134. [CrossRef] [PubMed]
14. Scott, I.A.; Attia, J.; Moynihan, R. Promises and perils of using genetic tests to predict risk of disease. *BMJ* **2020**, *368*, m14. [CrossRef]
15. Tluczek, A.; Laxova, A.; Grieve, A.; Heun, A.; Brown, R.L.; Rock, M.J.; Gershan, W.M.; Farrell, P.M. Long-term follow-up of cystic fibrosis newborn screening: Psychosocial functioning of adolescents and young adults. *J. Cyst. Fibros.* **2014**, *13*, 227–234. [CrossRef]
16. Farrell, M.H.; Farrell, P.M. Newborn screening for cystic fibrosis: Ensuring more good than harm. *J. Pediatr.* **2003**, *143*, 707–712. [CrossRef]
17. Sims, E.J.; Mugford, M.; Clark, A.; Aitken, D.; McCormick, J.; Mehta, G.; Mehta, A.; UK Cystic Fibrosis Database Steering Committee. Economic implications of newborn screening for cystic fibrosis: A cost of illness retrospective cohort study. *Lancet* **2007**, *369*, 1187–1195. [CrossRef]
18. Lewis, S.; Curnow, L.; Ross, M.; Massie, J. Parental attitudes to the identification of their infants as carriers of cystic fibrosis by newborn screening. *J. Paediatr. Child Health* **2006**, *42*, 533–537. [CrossRef]
19. Ulph, F.; Wright, S.; Dharni, N.; Payne, K.; Bennett, R.; Roberts, S.; Walshe, K.; Lavender, T. Provision of information about newborn screening antenatally: A sequential exploratory mixed-methods project. *Health Technol. Assess.* **2017**, *21*, 1–240. [CrossRef]
20. Ulph, F.; Cullinan, T.; Qureshi, N.; Kai, J. Parents' responses to receiving sickle cell or cystic fibrosis carrier results for their child following newborn screening. *Eur. J. Hum. Genet.* **2015**, *23*, 459–465. [CrossRef]
21. Ulph, F.; Cullinan, T.; Qureshi, N.; Kai, J. Informing children of their newborn screening carrier result for sickle cell or cystic fibrosis: Qualitative study of parents' intentions, views and support needs. *J. Genet. Couns.* **2014**, *23*, 409–420. [CrossRef] [PubMed]
22. Oliver, S.; Dezateux, C.; Kavanagh, J.; Lempert, T.; Stewart, R. Disclosing to parents newborn carrier status identified by routine blood spot screening. *Cochrane Database Syst. Rev.* **2004**, CD003859. [CrossRef] [PubMed]
23. Tluczek, A.; Orland, K.M.; Cavanagh, L. Psychosocial consequences of false-positive newborn screens for cystic fibrosis. *Qual. Health Res.* **2011**, *21*, 174–186. [CrossRef] [PubMed]
24. Tluczek, A.; Koscik, R.L.; Farrell, P.M.; Rock, M.J. Psychosocial risk associated with newborn screening for cystic fibrosis: Parents' experience while awaiting the sweat-test appointment. *Pediatrics* **2005**, *115*, 1692–1703. [CrossRef] [PubMed]
25. Kharrazi, M.; Yang, J.; Bishop, T.; Lessing, S.; Young, S.; Graham, S.; Pearl, M.; Chow, H.; Ho, T.; Gaffney, L.; et al. Newborn Screening for Cystic Fibrosis in California. *Pediatrics* **2015**, *136*, 1062–1072. [CrossRef]

26. Hayeems, R.Z.; Miller, F.A.; Vermeulen, M.; Potter, B.K.; Chakraborty, P.; Davies, C.; Carroll, J.C.; Ratjen, F.; Guttmann, A. False-positive newborn screening for cystic fibrosis and health care use. *Pediatrics* **2017**, *140*, e20170604. [CrossRef]
27. Beucher, J.; Leray, E.; Deneuville, E.; Roblin, M.; Pin, I.; Bremont, F.; Turck, D.; Giniès, J.-L.; Foucaud, P.; Derelle, J.; et al. Psychological effects of false-positive results in cystic fibrosis newborn screening: A two-year follow-up. *J. Pediatr.* **2010**, *156*, 771–776.e1. [CrossRef]
28. Castellani, C.; Duff, A.J.; Bell, S.C.; Heijerman, H.G.; Munck, A.; Ratjen, F.; Sermet-Gaudelus, I.; Southern, K.W.; Barben, J.; Hodková, P.; et al. ECFS best practice guidelines: The 2018 revision. *J. Cyst. Fibros.* **2018**, *17*, 153–178. [CrossRef]
29. Heeley, A.F.; Fagan, D.G. Trisomy 18, cystic fibrosis, and blood immunoreactive trypsin. *Lancet* **1984**, *1*, 169–170. [CrossRef]
30. Farrell, P.M.; White, T.B.; Ren, C.L.; Hempstead, S.E.; Accurso, F.; Derichs, N.; Howenstine, M.; McColley, S.A.; Rock, M.; Sermet-Gaudelus, I.; et al. Diagnosis of cystic fibrosis: Consensus guidelines from the cystic fibrosis foundation. *J. Pediatr.* **2017**, *181*, S4–S15.e1. [CrossRef]
31. Southern, K.W.; Barben, J.; Gartner, S.; Munck, A.; Castellani, C.; Mayell, S.J.; Davies, J.C.; Winters, V.; Murphy, J.; McColley, S.A.; et al. Inconclusive diagnosis after a positive newborn bloodspot screening result for cystic fibrosis; clarification of the harmonised international definition. *J. Cyst. Fibros.* **2019**, *18*, 778–780. [CrossRef] [PubMed]
32. Barben, J.; Castellani, C.; Dankert-Roelse, J.; Gartner, S.; Kashirskaya, N.; Linnane, B.; Mayell, S.; Munck, A.; Sands, D.; Pybus, S.; et al. The expansion and performance of national newborn screening programmes for cystic fibrosis in Europe. *J. Cyst. Fibros.* **2017**, *16*, 207–213. [CrossRef] [PubMed]
33. Munck, A.; Bourmaud, A.; Bellon, G.; Picq, P.; Farrell, P.M.; DPAM Study Group. Phenotype of children with inconclusive cystic fibrosis diagnosis after newborn screening. *Pediatr. Pulmonol.* **2020**. [CrossRef] [PubMed]
34. Munck, A.; Mayell, S.J.; Winters, V.; Shawcross, A.; Derichs, N.; Parad, R.; Barben, J.; Southern, K.W. Cystic Fibrosis Screen Positive, Inconclusive Diagnosis (CFSPID): A new designation and management recommendations for infants with an inconclusive diagnosis following newborn screening. *J. Cyst. Fibros.* **2015**, *14*, 706–713. [CrossRef] [PubMed]
35. Bombieri, C.; Claustres, M.; De Boeck, K.; Derichs, N.; Dodge, J.; Girodon, E.; Sermet, I.; Schwarz, M.; Tzetis, M.; Bareil, C.; et al. Recommendations for the classification of diseases as CFTR-related disorders. *J. Cyst. Fibros.* **2011**, *10* (Suppl. 2), S86–S102. [CrossRef]
36. Johnson, F.; Southern, K.W.; Ulph, F. Psychological impact on parents of an inconclusive diagnosis following newborn bloodspot screening for cystic fibrosis: A qualitative study. *Int. J. Neonat. Screen.* **2019**, *5*, 23. [CrossRef]
37. Castellani, C.; Southern, K.W.; Brownlee, K.; Roelse, J.D.; Duff, A.; Farrell, M.; Mehta, A.; Munck, A.; Pollitt, R.; Wilcken, B.; et al. European best practice guidelines for cystic fibrosis neonatal screening. *J. Cyst. Fibros.* **2009**, *8*, 153–173. [CrossRef]
38. Korzeniewski, S.J.; Young, W.I.; Hawkins, H.C.; Cavanagh, K.; Nasr, S.Z.; Langbo, C.; TenEyck, K.R.; Grosse, S.D.; Kleyn, M.; Grigorescu, V. Variation in immunoreactive trypsinogen concentrations among Michigan newborns and implications for cystic fibrosis newborn screening. *Pediatr. Pulmonol.* **2011**, *46*, 125–130. [CrossRef]
39. Bulent, K.; Memorial Ataşehir Hospital, İstanbul, Turkey; Refika, E.; Marmara University, Istanbul, Turkey. Personal Communication, 2020.
40. Munck, A.; Delmas, D.; Audrezet, M.P.; Lemonnier, L.; Cheillan, D.; Roussey, M. Optimization of the French cystic fibrosis newborn screening programme by a centralized tracking process. *J. Med. Screen.* **2018**, *25*, 6–12. [CrossRef]

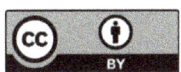

© 2020 by the authors. Licensee MDPI, Basel, Switzerland. This article is an open access article distributed under the terms and conditions of the Creative Commons Attribution (CC BY) license (http://creativecommons.org/licenses/by/4.0/).

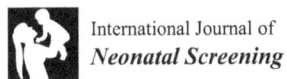

Review

Pancreatitis-Associated Protein in Neonatal Screening for Cystic Fibrosis: Strengths and Weaknesses

Olaf Sommerburg [1,2,*] and Jutta Hammermann [3]

[1] Division of Pediatric Pulmonology & Allergy and Cystic Fibrosis Center, Department of Pediatrics III, University of Heidelberg, Im Neuenheimer Feld 430, D-69120 Heidelberg, Germany
[2] Translational Lung Research Center Heidelberg (TLRC), Member of the German Center for Lung Research (DZL), Im Neuenheimer Feld 350, D-69120 Heidelberg, Germany
[3] Pediatric Department, University Hospital of Dresden, Fetscherstr. 74, D-01307 Dresden, Germany; Jutta.Hammermann@uniklinikum-dresden.de
* Correspondence: olaf.sommerburg@med.uni-heidelberg.de

Received: 4 February 2020; Accepted: 13 March 2020; Published: 30 March 2020

Abstract: There are currently four countries and one local region in Europe that use PAP in their newborn screening programme. The first country to employ PAP at a national level was the Netherlands, which started using IRT/PAP/DNA/EGA in 2011. Germany followed in 2016 with a slightly different IRT/PAP/DNA strategy. Portugal also started in 2016, but with an IRT/PAP/IRT programme, and in 2017, Austria changed its IRT/IRT protocol to an IRT/PAP/IRT program. In 2018, Catalonia started to use an IRT/PAP/IRT/DNA strategy. The strengths of PAP are the avoidance of carrier detection and a lower detection rate of CFSPID. PAP seems to have advantages in detecting CF in ethnically-diverse populations, as it is a biochemical approach to screening, which looks for pancreatic injury. Compared to an IRT/IRT protocol, an IRT/PAP protocol leads to earlier diagnoses. While PAP can be assessed with the same screening card as the first IRT, the second IRT in an IRT/IRT protocol requires a second heel prick around the 21st day of the patient's life. However, IRT/PAP has two main weaknesses. First, an IRT/PAP protocol seems to have a lower sensitivity compared to a well-functioning IRT/DNA protocol, and second, IRT/PAP that is performed as a purely biochemical protocol has a very low positive predictive value. However, if the advantages of PAP are to be exploited, a combination of IRT/PAP with genetic screening or a second IRT as a third tier could be an alternative for a sufficiently performing CF-NBS protocol.

Keywords: cystic fibrosis; newborn screening; biochemical screening; pancreatitis associated protein; immunoreactive trypsinogen

---

1. Introduction

Cystic Fibrosis Newborn screening (CF NBS) is widely accepted, but there is no universal screening strategy [1]. All programs start with a measurement of immunoreactive trypsinogen (IRT) in dried blood spots. As the second tier, a repeat measurement of the IRT concentration can be performed at the age of 2–3 weeks, but in the most common CF NBS protocols, IRT measurement as the first tier are combined with the search for population-specific *CFTR* mutations, which provides good sensitivity and specificity [2]. However, the use of *CFTR* mutation analysis is also associated with a few unsolved problems. For example, the detection of healthy carriers and of infants in whom the diagnosis of CF is inconclusive (CFSPID) is not the goal of CF NBS. Furthermore, with increasing migration in the world and the mixing of different ethnic groups, especially in big cities, there is a tendency in countries with genetic CF NBS to increase the number of *CFTR* mutations tested to ensure sufficient sensitivity. This leads to a further increase in the number of carriers and CFSPID. However, this makes information and counselling for families with children with CF, carriers, or CFSPID in these countries increasingly challenging [3,4]. In addition, in countries where informed consent for CF NBS is required, genetic CF NBS can significantly complicate the parental education and consent process.

In 1994, a French group suggested pancreatitis associated protein (PAP) as candidate for a marker for screening CF [5]. PAP is a secretory protein which is not measurable in blood under normal conditions, but which can be detected in high quantities in the context of pancreatic injury [6]. Two pilot studies showed that almost all IRT-negative newborns and most IRT-positive newborns without cystic fibrosis had normal PAP, while PAP was increased in newborns with CF [5,7]. Yet, the increase in PAP observed in newborns is not strictly CF-specific. If the measurement of PAP were used for CF NBS alone, it would have a similarly low specificity as the use of IRT alone. In the first French pilot studies, however, it was found that newborns with CF always had both an increased IRT and an increased PAP; in a further study, it was concluded that both parameters should be evaluated. The aim of this feasibility study was to compare the sensitivity and specificity of the combined measurement of IRT and PAP in the same neonatal population with the screening strategy (IRT/DNA/IRT) used in France at that time [8]. In this study, 204,748 newborns were included; the results published in 2005 showed that the performance of the IRT/PAP strategy was not inferior to that of the IRT/DNA/IRT strategy applied in parallel [8].

2. The Evolution of the PAP Kit

It is important to mention right at the beginning that the PAP kit has undergone several changes and improvements since it first appeared. For the data of the first publications on the use of PAP in CF NBS obtained from 1994 to 2003, an ELISA kit using a polyclonal antibody for antigen capture and detection was used [5,8,9]. When Sarles et al. published their lauded paper on the IRT/PAP protocol including recommended cut-offs in 2005 [8], the manufacturer (Dynabio, Marseille, France) had already changed the ELISA kit used for this evaluation, and the original kit, to which the recommendations referred, was no longer available. At that time, a new kit, called "MucoPAP", was available, which uses monoclonal antibodies to capture and detect antigens. Unfortunately, there were no new recommendations for the cut-off values for this MucoPAP kit to serve as guidelines. Thus, pilot studies that were later conducted in other European countries and which are described below used the cut-off values that were actually set with the previously-marketed kit. The new cut-off recommendations for the MucoPAP kit with the monoclonal antibody were published by Sarles et al., but not before 2014 [10]. In the meantime, however, results from other European pilot studies had been published [11–13]. Some had used different cut-off values in their protocols or had used different safety net strategies to ensure sufficient sensitivity [11,12,14]. During the pilot study in the Netherlands, which will be discussed below [12], the researchers realized that the dilution factor recommended in the product description of the manufacturer of the MucoPAP kit for calculating the measured values after comparison with the reference standard was incorrect. After contact with Dynabio, this was officially corrected, but this meant that the originally recommended cut-off values had to be corrected by a factor of 1.67. To avoid further confusion for the reader, we will mention from now on in this review only the values with the corrected dilution factors, but we will add the noncorrected values in parenthesis, if these values were used in the respective original articles (e.g., in [8,11,13]).

From 2013 onwards, a further version of the PAP-ELISA, the MucoPAP-F-Kit, was available from DynaBio, which uses an alternative readout system. With this kit, the antigen–antibody complexes are detected by a streptavidin–europium conjugate, which serves as fluorescence enhancement solution. This makes it possible to detect highly fluorescent chelates that emit at 620 nm when excited at 337 nm. Compared to measurements with the MucoPAP kit with photometric detection, the MucoPAP-F kit seems to be much more stable and has a higher reproducibility. It is important to note that the cut-off values of PAP measurements with MucoPAP and MucoPAP-F are not directly comparable.

In 2016, Dynabio launched a new version of its PAP kit with photometric detection, the "MucoPAP II". The company claimed that this test had a much better intraspot reproducibility of ranges and controls compared to the previous MucoPAP kit, but the calculations from the new ranges were ~1.5 times lower than with the old kit. As a result, the PAP cut-off values had to be changed again, as done for the Austrian CF NBS in 2017.

Unfortunately, the different PAP cut-off values published over the years have meant that publications on the performance of PAP-based CF-NBS protocols are very difficult to compare.

3. Description of Selected European Pilot Studies

In 2005, Sarles et al. published their study, which demonstrated the feasibility of using PAP in conjunction with IRT [8]. While IRT and PAP were measured in parallel during the study, after an evaluation, the authors proposed a protocol in which IRT is used as the first tier and PAP as the second, which is only performed in case of increased IRT. In this respect, the so-called IRT/PAP protocol was very similar to the IRT/IRT and IRT/DNA protocols known before. In the protocol proposed by Sarles et al., a fixed IRT cut-off value of 50 µg/L was used to ensure sufficient sensitivity. For PAP, two IRT-dependent cut-off values were proposed to reduce the number of newborns with CFSPID and improve the positive predictive value (PPV): If IRT was measured between 50.0–99.9 µg/L, a PAP cut-off value of 3.0 (before correction of the dilution factor 1.8) µg/L should have been applied; if IRT was > 100 µg/L, a PAP cut-off of 1.67 (before correction of the dilution factor 1.0) µg/L should have been used [8] (Figure 1A). This protocol was the starting point for all changes that were later made in other CF NBS protocols based on PAP.

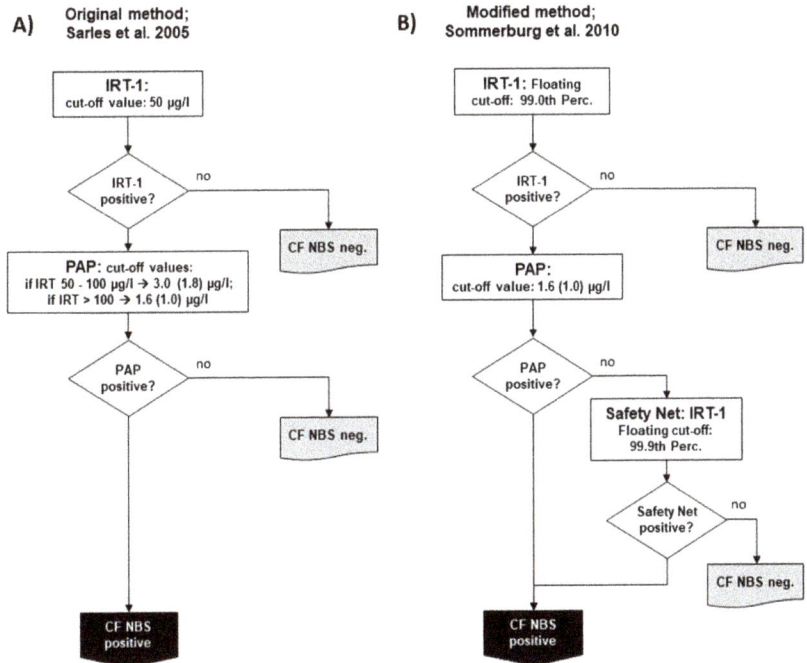

Figure 1. Schemes of the two main variants of the pure biochemical IRT/PAP protocol: (**A**) IRT/PAP protocol published by Sarles et al. 2005 [8] and (**B**) the IRT/PAP-SN protocol with IRT-dependent safety net modified by Sommerburg et al. [11]. Values in parenthesis show the PAP cut-off values as given before correction of the dilution factor by the manufacturer (see explanation in the main Text).

After the publication of this study in 2005, many specialists involved in CF NBS were interested in PAP as a new biochemical parameter and as an alternative to genetic CF screening. Although IRT/DNA protocols became the gold standard for CF NBS in terms of sensitivity and PPV, they had the disadvantages described above. However, if IRT/PAP is used as a pure biochemical protocol, the detection of healthy carriers can be completely avoided. This was the reason why studies were started in several countries around the world in the following years to verify the results of the French study and to adapt the method to local requirements. Unfortunately, not all the results of these studies were published. To the best of our knowledge, data are currently available only from France [10], Germany [11,15], The Netherlands [12,16], Czech Republic [13] and Portugal [17].

In 2008, new pilot studies started in the Netherlands and Germany. In the study in the Netherlands, samples from 145,499 newborns were measured using the slightly modified IRT/PAP protocol proposed by Sarles et al. [8], and the results were compared with those of an IRT/DNA/EGA protocol [12]. In the modified IRT/PAP protocol, the IRT cut-off used was set at 60 instead of 50 µg/L. Furthermore, the photometric measurement of the commercially available MucoPAP kit (Dynabio, Marseille, France) was replaced by a flouroimmunoassay using a Streptavidin-Europium tracer for the detection of PAP in a manner that is similar to that later introduced in the MucoPAP-F kit. The two IRT dependent PAP cut-offs were performed as follows: a positive result for PAP was defined if IRT was ≥ 100 µg/L and PAP was ≥ 1.6 µg/L or IRT was ≥ 60 µg/L and PAP was ≥ 3.0 µg/L. In the IRT/DNA protocol, the *CFTR* gene was sequenced (extended gene analysis, EGA) if, in an initial search with a panel of 35 *CFTR* mutations, none or only one *CFTR* mutation was found. In a post hoc analysis, a combination of both strategies (IRT/PAP/DNA(35)/EGA) was shown to be the best compromise for the requirements of the CF NBS program in the Netherlands.

In Germany, separate pilot studies were started in 2008 in two NBS centres (Dresden and Heidelberg) and continued until the start of the nationwide CF NBS programme in 2016. However, it should be mentioned that preliminary IRT/PAP trials had already been carried out in the CF NBS centre Dresden since 2005. The IRT/PAP protocol there was performed as originally described by Sarles et al. [8,14], but, as in the Netherlands, the ELISA MucoPAP kit (Dynabio, Marseille, France) was used for PAP quantification, and the photometric detection was replaced by fluorometric measurements [14]. Every year, 18,000 newborns are examined in Dresden and 110,000 in Heidelberg. In Heidelberg, however, less than half of the hospitals that send Guthrie cards to the NBS centre participated in the CF NBS pilot study. The IRT/PAP strategy in Heidelberg has been modified by applying a floating cut-off for IRT using the 99.0th percentile, which is often used in other CF NBS protocols. For PAP, the Heidelberg protocol relied only on one PAP cut-off using the lower PAP cut-off of the two IRT-dependent PAP cut-offs of the original protocol by Sarles et al. [8], which was defined at ≥ 1.67 µg/L (before correction of the dilution factor ≥ 1.0 µg/L) (Figure 1B). In both Dresden and Heidelberg, a safety net strategy was applied from the first year of the study due to ongoing discussions about the possibility of low sensitivity when using PAP. According to this, CF NBS was positive when the IRT ≥ was 99.9 percentile, regardless of the PAP value, which was measured as 2nd tier test. From 2008 until 2016 in Heidelberg, but not in Dresden, a genetic CF NBS protocol searching for the four most common *CFTR* mutations in Germany (IRT/DNA (4)) was run in parallel as a reference.

In 2009, another pilot study was started in the Czech Republic (Prague). In this prospective study 106,522 newborns from Bohemia, the western region of the Czech Republic, were examined to compare the IRT/PAP protocol, as originally published by Sarles et al. [8], with an IRT/DNA/IRT protocol that had been started two years earlier. While for the IRT/PAP protocol the same IRT and PAP cut-offs values were used as originally published, for the IRT/DNA/IRT protocol, the initial IRT was rated positive when the value was ≥ 65 µg/L. The initial DNA test included 32 CFTR mutations, while from July 2010, it contained 50 CFTR mutations, which represented 90.8% and 92.8% of all CFTR mutations of Czech CF patients, respectively. The results of these two protocols were compared and used to simulate an IRT/PAP/DNA(50) protocol, whose performance was then compared to that of the IRT/PAP and IRT/DNA(50)/IRT protocol.

Some of the questions concerning the PAP-based CF NBS protocols could only be answered through cooperation and combinations of study results, as done with those from Heidelberg, Dresden, and Prague. This was the only way to answer questions about the initial IRT cut-off value, the PAP cut-off values, the need for an IRT-dependent safety net, and the performance of a CF NBS strategy using the product of the IRT and PAP values [14,18].

Another PAP-based CF NBS study with 255,000 newborns started in Portugal at the end of 2013 [17]. To the best of our knowledge, this study was the first to test an IRT/PAP/IRT strategy. The cut-off value of the initial IRT was first set at 50 µg/L, but was increased to 65 µg/L after only four months. The second IRT measurement as a third stage strategy was either performed when the initial IRT ≥ was 150 µg/L (SN strategy), the PAP ≥ was 0.5 and the IRT was between 100 and 150 µg/L, or the PAP was ≥ 1.6 µg/L. For PAP analysis, the MucoPAP-F kit (Dynabio, Marseille, France) was used.

4. Findings from the Pilot Studies

4.1. IRT/PAP Protocols Detect Less Healthy Carriers

The obvious advantage of an IRT/PAP strategy is the complete avoidance of the detection of healthy carriers of *CFTR* mutations by using the pure biochemical parameters IRT and PAP. Interestingly, however, the published results from the Netherlands, Heidelberg (Germany), and the Czech Republic also showed that only 10–20% of newborns who tested positive in IRT/PAP were healthy carriers [11–13]. This shows that the heterozygous presence of a *CFTR* mutation alone does not lead to an increased PAP value in the majority of cases, which, in turn, excludes a direct dependence on the presence of certain *CFTR* mutations. This fact may seem unimportant at first glance, but it is of considerable relevance when the decision has to be made in countries with very heterogeneous ethnic populations about whether a genetic or a biochemical CF NBS should be used. While an increased number of *CFTR* mutations in the panel of an IRT/DNA protocol inevitably also increases the number of healthy carriers, a significantly lower detection rate of carriers can be achieved by adding a PAP test prior to the search for *CFTR* mutations. In the pilot study in the Netherlands, the reduction of carriers by the IRT/PAP/DNA(35)/EGA strategy was 88% in comparison to the IRT/DNA (35)/EGA strategy [12].

4.2. IRT/PAP Protocols Detect Less CFSPID

The notion that PAP-based CF NBS protocols detect less CFSPID was primarily based on the fact that the first IRT/PAP protocol by Sarles et al., with its two IRT-dependent PAP cut-off levels, was designed in a way that the majority of CFSPID patients are not detected [8]. The reason for using this design was based on the assumption that in the IRT range from 50.0 to 99.9 µg/L, lower PAP values could reflect mild CF phenotypes that are not the goal of CF NBS. As expected, those IRT/PAP protocols showed also in the following pilot studies a significantly lower detection rate of newborns with CFSPID [12,13]. However, so far, there is no evidence that the PAP concentration generally correlates with the severity of CF disease. This fact is also supported by data from the other pilot studies showing higher PAP concentrations in CFSPID or patients with *CFTR* mutations leading to pancreatic sufficiency and low PAP concentrations in some patients with *CFTR* mutations leading to pancreatic insufficiency and a severe CF phenotype (e.g., [18]). When the pilot study on the IRT/PAP strategy was started in Heidelberg in 2008, it was decided that only a single PAP cut-off level of ≥ 1.67 µg/L (before correction of the dilution factor 1.0 µg/L) [11] should be used. Nevertheless, even with this protocol, a significantly lower detection rate for newborns with CFSPID was found. While only 1.6% of the children positively screened by the IRT/PAP protocol with subsequent detection of 2 *CFTR* mutations were newborns with CFSPID, the rate with the IRT/DNA [4] protocol run in parallel was 7.3% [18]. These results indicate that a CF NBS with PAP alone can reduce the detection of CFSPID.

4.3. IRT/PAP Protocols May Show Lower Sensitivity than IRT/DNA Protocols

The published pilot studies by Sarles et al. showed that the IRT/PAP strategy had the same—if not better—sensitivity than the IRT/DNA(20/30)/IRT protocol conducted in parallel [8,10]. However, these results could not really be confirmed in any of the other pilot studies (e.g., [12,13,15]). However, it turned out that there may be a variety of reasons for possible reductions of the sensitivity of an

IRT/PAP protocol. Several of these drawbacks were addressed in the pilot studies, and it became clear that some of them could be overcome by minor protocol changes. Nevertheless, most of the sensitivity improvements proposed below are at the expense of the PPV, another important quality criterion of CF-NBS protocols.

1. *The use of an IRT-dependent safety net:* When the pilot studies were started in the Germany, the general concern was that the PAP strategy had a worse sensitivity than a well-performing genetic CF NBS. Similar to the IRT/DNA protocols with a restricted mutation panel, an IRT-dependent safety net was added six months after starting the pilot studies. Therefore, CF NBS is considered positive if the initial IRT is above the 99.9th percentile, regardless of the PAP result. When the results of the pilot study conducted in Prague (Czech Republic) were published in 2012, the IRT/PAP strategy showed a very low sensitivity of only 76% [13]. After a re-evaluation for a joint, posthoc analysis of the raw data from Prague, Dresden and Heidelberg, it was found that the sensitivity of the Prague PAP-based CF NBS would have been 89.5% if the colleagues there had used the original IRT/PAP protocol but with the IRT-dependent safety net, as was done in the German centres [18]. Furthermore, a recently published paper on the Dutch CF NBS shows that out of eight CF patients not detected in the IRT/PAP part of the IRT/PAP/DNA(35)/EGA strategy, five would probably have been found if such an IRT-dependent safety net had been used [16].

2. *Renouncing the two IRT-dependent PAP cut-off values:* As mentioned, the reason to use the two IRT-dependent PAP cut-offs was based on the assumption that such a protocol would avoid the detection of CFSPID. In addition, IRT/PAP protocols with two IRT-dependent PAP cut-off values were proposed to detect less healthy newborns as false positives compared to protocols with only one PAP cut-off value. However, the results of the aforementioned joint posthoc analysis of the data from Prague, Dresden, and Heidelberg suggest that IRT/PAP protocols with two IRT-dependent PAP cut-off values may have limited sensitivity compared to those with only one PAP cut-off value. In a joint simulation of raw data from Prague and Heidelberg, it was found that by using two PAP cut-off values, four newborns with two mutations in the *CFTR* gene would have been missed, but would have been detected by the protocol with one PAP cut-off. Only one out of these four newborns carried a *CFTR* mutation with varying clinical consequence and had a normal sweat chloride. The other three newborns were diagnosed with classical CF with pancreatic insufficiency. Two out of these three CF patients suffered from MI and would have been diagnosed clinically. However, the third CF patient would have been missed by all IRT/PAP protocols relying on two IRT-dependent PAP cut-offs [18]. It can be argued whether one has to consider three missed patients with CF or only one, since two out of these three presented with MI.

3. Anyway, the fact that newborns carrying two CF-causing mutations were not detected due to the IRT/PAP protocol with two PAP cut-offs raises the question of whether such a protocol can achieve sufficient sensitivity. It is interesting to note that if the colleagues in Prague had used the same IRT/PAP protocol as that used in Heidelberg, not only with the IRT dependent safety net, but also with only one PAP cut-off value, the sensitivity would have been 94.7%. Also, in a recently published work on the aforementioned Dutch CF NBS program, it was shown that if only one PAP cut-off value had been used, one CF patient out of the eight CF patients not found would still have been detected. With the five CF patients that would have been found by the safety Net, six of the eight CF patients would have been found [16].

4. *Lowering of PAP cut-off values:* Due to the fact that all the pilot studies mentioned above were started with a MucoPAP kit whose PAP cut-off values had not yet been sufficiently evaluated, the most obvious solution for sensitivity problems would have been to simply adjust the PAP cut-off values downwards. Actually, this was also done later by Sarles et al. and reported in a publication in 2014 [10]. However, significantly lowered PAP cut-off values were not only found there, but were seen in recent years also in other PAP-based protocols (e.g., [17]). Yet, it is precisely this approach that significantly increases the number of false-positive newborns detected.

5. *Using both biochemical markers, IRT and PAP, at the same time:* In all current PAP-based CF-NBS protocols, IRT and PAP are used sequentially. However, the simultaneous use of both biomarkers instead of two steps, e.g., by using the product of IRT and PAP, has the potential to make the screening strategy significantly more sensitive than in the IRT/PAP protocols currently in use. Despite the simultaneous use of both parameters, IRT can still be used as a first-tier-parameter that triggers the PAP measurement if it is above a certain cut-off value. Such an approach was demonstrated by the Dresden group in a posthoc analysis using raw data from the pilot studies of the two German CF NBS centres, i.e., Dresden and Heidelberg [14]. The data from Heidelberg showed the highest sensitivity with the IRTxPAP product (98.3%), in contrast to the revised strategy of Sarles et al. published in 2014 (94.9%), and also in contrast to the Heidelberg IRT/PAP-SN protocol (96.6%).

6. *Time-dependent sampling of the dried blood for neonatal screening:* There is unpublished local experience from Australia, still acknowledged by a number of CF NBS specialists, that the use of PAP is not sensitive enough if the dried blood sample for NBS is taken from the infant before the age of 48 h. As a reason for this, it was assumed that the PAP blood levels in infants with cystic fibrosis increase over time. According to our experience, this could be true, but not only in CF infants. In Germany, the collection of the dried blood sample is usually carried out between the 36th and 72nd hour of life, but for special reasons, we sometimes see early or late sampling. If we group all available PAP values of the infants studied in recent years into 12-h intervals, we see a trend of an increase in the 25th, 50th, and 75th percentiles from 24 h to 72 h (personal communication O. Sommerburg). However, when we focused on CF patients not found in our IRT/PAP protocol, we could not confirm that these CF patients were missed because the time of collection of the dry blood sample was before the 48th hour of life. In this regard, after more than 10 years of PAP-based CF NBS, we consider it to be proven that PAP screening with samples collected between 36 and 48 h of life is feasible. Yet, if the majority of infants in a country are screened for NBS before the 36th hour of life, we might imagine that PAP blood levels might still be too low. In this case, we would recommend a comprehensive pilot study to test the feasibility of a PAP-based CF NBS also under these conditions.

4.4. Pure Biochemical IRT/PAP Protocols Show a Relatively Low Positive Predictive Value

The reason why no current PAP-based CF-NBS screening program uses a purely biochemical IRT/PAP strategy has to do with the associated low PPV. In various publications from the pilot studies mentioned above, the PPV was stated to be 7.8–15.3% [12–15]. Furthermore, it is remarkable that almost all of the aforementioned interventions to improve the sensitivity of the PAP step in an IRT/PAP strategy lead to a further reduction of the PPV. However, it should be noted that the disadvantage of a higher false positive rate is compensated for by the expected higher sensitivity. Of note, also a DNA-based protocol, especially with a limited *CFTR* mutation panel, does not guarantee that the required PPV of 30% is reached, as seen with the IRT/DNA protocol run in parallel in the CF-NBS centre Heidelberg (15.3%) and in the French study published 2014 (27.1%) [10,15] (Table 1). However, the combination of a PAP-based two-tier protocol with a third step test such as a search for *CFTR* mutations or a second IRT will maintain the higher sensitivity but eliminate the disadvantage of the lower PPV. This is the reason why all CF NBS protocols currently in use are based on PAP three- or even four-tier strategies. In DNA-based CF-NBS strategies today, extended gene analysis is often used as the 3rd step after the 2nd step was performed with a limited CFTR mutation panel. This strategy also improves both the sensitivity and the PPV of the protocol. However, it does detect significantly more newborns with CFSPID, which is not really desirable. In this respect, a well-performing IRT/PAP/DNA protocol would be superior to a genetic protocol, as described above.

Table 1. Performance indicators sensitivity (%), positive predictive value (PPV, (%)) and CF/CFSPID ratio of a number of representative genetic and PAP-based CF-NBS protocols of different countries and regions compared to the ECFS standard. The numbers in parentheses within the protocol name reflect the CFTR mutations in the panel used.

2nd Tier Test	Reference	Protocol	Region/Country	n Screened	Prevalence of CF	Sensitivity (%) w/o MI	PPV (%)
	ECFS standard [19]					≥95	≥30
IRT	Calvin et al. 2012 [20]	IRT/IRT	East Anglia (UK)	582,966	1:2286	93.8	67.3
DNA	Calvin et al. 2012 [20]	IRT/DNA(29)/IRT	East Anglia (UK)	147,764	1:2111	90.2	85.9
	Sommerburg et al. 2015 [15]	IRT/DNA(4)+SN	Southwest Germany	252,020	1:4582	95.1	15.3
	Kharrazi et al. 2015 [21]	IRT/DNA(28–40)/EGA	California	2,573,293	1:6899	92	34
	Sontag et al. 2016 [22]	IRT/IRT/DNA(41–48)	Colorado, Wyoming, Texas	1,520,079	1:5548	96.2	19.7
	Lundman et al. 2016 [23]	IRT/DNA/EGA	Norway	181,859	1:8660	95	43
	Skov et al. [24]	IRT/DNA(1)/EGA	Denmark	126,338	1:4866	91.7	84.6
PAP	Sommerburg et al. 2015 [15]	IRT/PAP+SN	Southwest Germany and East-Saxony (Germany)	328,176	1:4860	96.0	8.8
	Weidler et al. [14]	IRTxPAP	Southwest Germany and East-Saxony (Germany)	410,111	1:5258	97.4	8.2
	Marcao et al. 2018 [17]	IRT/PAP/IRT	Portugal	255,000	1:7500	94.4	41.3
	Dankert-Roelse et al. 2019 [16]	IRT/PAP/DNA(35)/EGA	The Netherlands	819,879	1:6029	90	63

4.5. Current PAP-Based CF Screening Protocols in Use

Today, PAP-based CF NS protocols may achieve sufficient performance. One strength of a PAP-based CF NBS is the possibility to use it in multiethnic populations where an appropriate genetic screening is either not possible or is too cost-intensive. Table 1 gives an overview of the performance of PAP-based protocols compared to selected purely biochemical IRT/IRT- or genetic CF NBS protocols. There are currently five European countries where a CF NBS strategy based on PAP is used either in a national or regional setting.

The Netherlands: The first country to use PAP at nationwide level after a pilot study [12] was the Netherlands, which started its national screening program with an IRT/PAP/DNA(35)/EGA protocol in 2011 [16] (Figure 2A). The program started using the commercially-available MucoPAP kit (Dynabio, Marseille, France), but, as mentioned above, the photometric measurement was replaced by a flouroimmunoassay during the pilot study. Until 2016, the IRT/PAP part of the protocol was performed as proposed by Sarles et al. [8], except for the increased IRT cut-off values (now 60 μg/L). However, after the last evaluation published in 2019 [16], the IRT/PAP part of the screening protocol was changed in two points. Firstly, the lower of the two PAP cut-off values was reduced, and secondly, a safety net was introduced for the PAP step, which is based on the 99.9th IRT percentile, as in the protocol according to Sommerburg et al. [11,18]. It may be expected that this variant of the CF-NBS protocol will now have a very high sensitivity and a very good PPV. So far, however, there are no newly-published data on this.

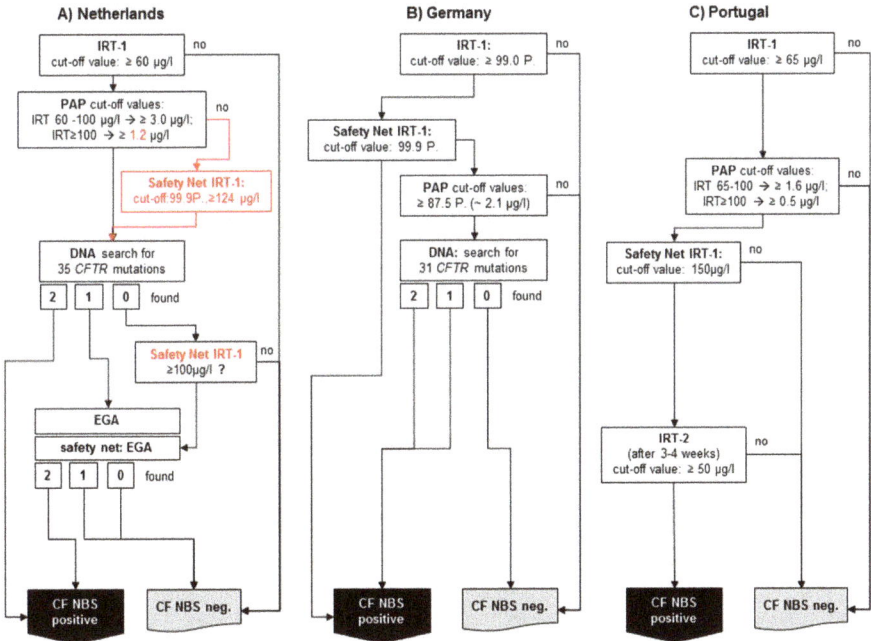

Figure 2. Simplified schemes of three selected PAP-based CF NBS protocols currently used: (**A**) The Netherlands: IRT/PAP/DNA(35)/EGA protocol including last modifications from 2016, (**B**) Germany: IRT/PAP-SN/DNA(31) protocol, (**C**) Portugal: IRT/PAP-SN/IRT protocol.

To the best of our knowledge, after the MucoPAP-F became commercially available, it was used for this program. However, it should be noted that in the Netherlands, the two IRT-dependent PAP cut-offs as proposed by Sarles (IRT ≥ 100 μg/L: PAP cut-off ≥ 1.6 μg/L and IRT 60–100 μg/L: PAP cut-off ≥ 3.0 μg/L) were maintained, although it has been recognised that the fluorometric read-out of

MucoPAP is higher than that with photometric detection. Nevertheless, this is not a disadvantage for the overall performance. In the genetic part of the protocol, an initial screen will be performed with 35 *CFTR* mutations. Following a different procedure in the past, there is, today, a very comprehensive genetic approach (Figure 2A). All samples showing only 1 *CFTR* mutation and those without mutation but with an IRT > 100 (safety net) receive a very high level extensive gene analysis. Nevertheless, the overall sensitivity of the protocol in the evaluated five years is only 90%, which does not meet the criteria of the ECFS standards of care [19]. The reason for this is clearly the IRT/PAP part and not the DNA (35)/EGA part of the protocol. As shown by Dankert-Roelse et al. 2019 [16] (given also in Table 1), seven CF patients were missed by a low IRT and eight by a low PAP. While problems with a low IRT are difficult to circumvent, the majority of CF patients missed by PAP, as described above, might have been found if a protocol like the one according to Sommerburg et al. [11,18] or Weidler et al. [14] had been used.

In Germany, a PAP-based protocol with a DNA analysis as third tier is also used (Figure 2B). The IRT/PAP-SN part follows the recommendations of Sommerburg et al. 2014, and contains a floating IRT cut-off at the 99.0th percentile and only one PAP cut-off value. Originally, the lower PAP cut-off value (1.6 µg/L) according to Sarles et al. 2005 was used; however, the recommendation is now to apply the 87.5th PAP percentile calculated from PAP values of a nonpreselected population of newborns [25].

After the introduction of the new MucoPAP-F-Kit, the PAP cut-off value, e.g., at the CF NBS centre Heidelberg, is 2.1 µg/L.

If a sample is PAP positive, a search for the 31 most common disease-causing *CFTR* mutations detected by the German national register will be done. If one or two CFTR mutations are found, the sample is rated CF NBS positive. Also, the IRT-dependent safety net (IRT ≥ 99.9th percentile) is used. While samples whose IRT is between 99.0 and 99.9th percentile will be tested for PAP and DNA, samples with an IRT ≥ 99.9th percentile will be immediately rated CF NBS positive [25]. As a reason for this decision, the authorities argued that CF patients whose CFTR mutations were not included in the panel should not be discriminated on the basis of their origin. The expected PPV was calculated in a post hoc analysis and was expected to be 20%, which would not meet the European standards of care [19,26]. This kind of IRT-dependent safety net remains questionable also for other reasons. For example, there is currently no modern CF NBS protocol in which a sample is considered positive after an ultra-high IRT alone. Furthermore, it was shown that, as previously expected, only about 25% of CF patients diagnosed with this protocol received a search for *CFTR* mutations during the CF NBS protocol [26]. Based on data from the Heidelberg IRT/PAP+SN pilot study, the sensitivity of the protocol was estimated to be 96% in the post hoc analysis mentioned above [26]. A complete evaluation of the CF NBS protocol used in Germany is now scheduled to be conducted after 3 years of application.

Portugal started in 2016 with an IRT/PAP-SN/IRT protocol which was evaluated before in the aforementioned pilot study (Figure 2C) [17]. To the best of our knowledge, there are currently no changes in the protocol. The IRT cut-off level was set at 65 µg/L. PAP is measured with the Muco PAP F kit. The PAP cut-off values are IRT dependent: If the IRT value is between 65 and 100 µg/L, a PAP cut-off value of ≥ 1.6 µg/L applies, with an IRT value of ≥ 100 µg/L a PAP cut-off value of ≥ 0.5 applies. Furthermore, an IRT SN strategy (≥150 µg/L) also triggers the measurement of a second IRT (50 µg/L). In our opinion, the PAP cut-off values seem rather low considering the fluorimetric readout of the MucoPAP-F kit used. However, this approach may be advantageous for the sensitivity of the protocol with regard to the multiethnic population in Portugal, especially since the second IRT measurement in IRT/PAP positive neonates will achieve a PPV as required by the European standards. In the pilot study the sensitivity was 94.4% and the PPV 41.03% [17].

In 2017, Austria changed from an IRT/IRT to an IRT/PAP-SN/IRT protocol. PAP measurement is done with the MucoPAP II kit. For the initial IRT, a cut-off value of 65 ng/L was set. The PAP measurement is based on Sarles et al. with two IRT-dependent PAP cut-off values [8,10] that were adapted to the conditions of MucoPAP II: If IRT is between 65 and 100 µg/L, a PAP cut-off value of ≥ 2.5 µg/L applies, if IRT is ≥ 100 µg/L, a PAP cut-off value of ≥ 1.33 µg/L is valid. In addition an

IRT-dependent SN (IRT ≥ 130 µg/L) is used. Both an increased PAP and an ultra-high IRT (SN) trigger the second IRT (sampled after 3–4 weeks of age, cut-off value 50 µg/L) [27].

In 2018, Catalonia started using an IRT/PAP-SN/IRT/DNA strategy. PAP measurement is done with the MucoPAP-F kit. The initial IRT cut-off value was set at 50 ng/L. For the second tier, two IRT-dependent PAP cut-off values [8,10] are used, but with other cut-off values, as published elsewhere: If IRT is between 50 and 80 µg/L, a PAP cut-off value of ≥ 1.95 µg/L is used, if IRT is ≥ 80 µg/L, a PAP cut-off value of ≥ 1.0 µg/L applies. An IRT dependent SN with an IRT cut-off value of ≥ 130 µg/L was also implemented in Catalonia. Both an increased PAP and an ultra-high IRT (SN) trigger the second IRT (sampled after 21–30 days of life, IRT cut-off value 35 µg/L). If the second IRT is positive, a comprehensive genetic analysis is performed [28].

Of the PAP-based CF NBS protocols currently used in a national or regional screening programme, only the Netherlands has so far provided performance data of sufficient quality [16]. It is obvious that the data from the other programmes must also be evaluated without delay and the results published. PAP-based protocols definitely have advantages in multiethnic populations, and help to detect less carriers and CFSPID. While the problem of a too low PPV caused by purely biochemical IRT/PAP protocols is probably no longer relevant, as currently, only protocols with at least three tiers are in use, the problem of sufficient sensitivity remains of high relevance.

Funding: This research received no external funding.

Conflicts of Interest: The authors declare no conflict of interest.

References

1. Castellani, C.; Southern, K.W.; Brownlee, K.; Roelse, J.D.; Duff, A.; Farrell, M.; Mehta, A.; Munck, A.; Pollitt, R.; Sermet-Gaudelus, I.; et al. European best practice guidelines for cystic fibrosis neonatal screening. *J. Cyst. Fibros.* **2009**, *8*, 153–173. [CrossRef] [PubMed]
2. Wilcken, B.M.; Wiley, V. Newborn screening methods for cystic fibrosis. *Paediatr. Respir. Rev.* **2003**, *4*, 272–277. [CrossRef]
3. Munck, A.; Delmas, M.; Audrézet, M.-P.; Lemonnier, L.; Cheillan, D.; Roussey, M. Optimization of the French cystic fibrosis newborn screening programme by a centralized tracking process. *J. Med Screen.* **2017**, *25*, 6–12. [CrossRef] [PubMed]
4. Terlizzi, V.; Mergni, G.; Buzzetti, R.; Centrone, C.; Zavataro, L.; Braggion, C. Cystic fibrosis screen positive inconclusive diagnosis (CFSPID): Experience in Tuscany, Italy. *J. Cyst. Fibros.* **2019**, *18*, 484–490. [CrossRef] [PubMed]
5. Iovanna, J.L.; Férec, C.; Sarles, J.; Dagorn, J.C. The pancreatitis-associated protein (PAP). A new candidate for neonatal screening of cystic fibrosis. *Comptes Rendus de l'Académie des Sciences Series III Sciences de la Vie* **1994**, *317*, 561–564.
6. Iovanna, J.L.; Keim, V.; Nordback, I.; Montalto, G.; Camarena, J.; Letoublon, C.; Levy, P.; Berthézène, P.; Dagorn, J.-C. Serum levels of pancreatitis-associated protein as indicators of the course of acute pancreatitis. *Gastroenterology* **1994**, *106*, 728–734. [CrossRef]
7. Sarles, J.; Barthellemy, S.; Férec, C.; Iovanna, J.; Roussey, M.; Farriaux, J.-P.; Toutain, A.; Berthelot, J.; Maurin, N.; Codet, J.-P.; et al. Blood concentrations of pancreatitis associated protein in neonates: Relevance to neonatal screening for cystic fibrosis. *Arch. Dis. Child. Fetal Neonatal Ed.* **1999**, *80*, F118–F122. [CrossRef] [PubMed]
8. Sarles, J.; Berthézène, P.; Le Louarn, C.; Somma, C.; Perini, J.-M.; Catheline, M.; Mirallié, S.; Luzet, K.; Roussey, M.; Farriaux, J.-P.; et al. Combining Immunoreactive Trypsinogen and Pancreatitis-Associated Protein Assays, a Method of Newborn Screening for Cystic Fibrosis that Avoids DNA Analysis. *J. Pediatr.* **2005**, *147*, 302–305. [CrossRef] [PubMed]
9. Barthellemy, S.; Maurin, N.; Roussey, M.; Férec, C.; Murolo, S.; Berthézène, P.; Iovanna, J.L.; Dagorn, J.C.; Sarles, J. Evaluation of 47,213 infants in neonatal screening for cystic fibrosis, using pancreatitis-associated protein and immunoreactive trypsinogen assays. *Arch. Pédiatrie* **2001**, *8*, 275–281. [CrossRef]

10. Sarles, J.; Giorgi, R.; Berthézène, P.; Munck, A.; Cheillan, D.; Dagorn, J.-C.; Roussey, M. Neonatal screening for cystic fibrosis: Comparing the performances of IRT/DNA and IRT/PAP. *J. Cyst. Fibros.* **2014**, *13*, 384–390. [CrossRef] [PubMed]
11. Sommerburg, O.; Lindner, M.; Muckenthaler, M.; Kohlmueller, D.; Leible, S.; Feneberg, R.; Kulozik, A.E.; Mall, M.A.; Hoffmann, G.F. Initial evaluation of a biochemical cystic fibrosis newborn screening by sequential analysis of immunoreactive trypsinogen and pancreatitis-associated protein (IRT/PAP) as a strategy that does not involve DNA testing in a Northern European population. *J. Inherit. Metab. Dis.* **2010**, *33*, 263–271. [CrossRef] [PubMed]
12. Langen, A.M.M.V.-V.; Loeber, J.G.; Elvers, B.; Triepels, R.H.; Gille, J.J.; Van Der Ploeg, C.P.B.; Reijntjens, S.; Dompeling, E.; Dankert-Roelse, J.E. Novel strategies in newborn screening for cystic fibrosis: A prospective controlled study. *Thorax* **2012**, *67*, 289–295. [CrossRef] [PubMed]
13. Krulisova, V.; Balaščaková, M.; Skalická, V.; Piskackova, T.; Holubova, A.; Paděrová, J.; Krenkova, P.; Dvořáková, L.; Zemkova, D.; Kracmar, P.; et al. Prospective and parallel assessments of cystic fibrosis newborn screening protocols in the Czech Republic: IRT/DNA/IRT versus IRT/PAP and IRT/PAP/DNA. *Eur. J. Nucl. Med. Mol. Imaging* **2012**, *171*, 1223–1229.
14. Weidler, S.; Stopsack, K.H.; Hammermann, J.; Sommerburg, O.; Mall, M.A.; Hoffmann, G.F.; Kohlmüller, D.; Okun, J.G.; Macek, M.; Votava, F.; et al. A product of immunoreactive trypsinogen and pancreatitis-associated protein as second-tier strategy in cystic fibrosis newborn screening. *J. Cyst. Fibros.* **2016**, *15*, 752–758. [CrossRef] [PubMed]
15. Sommerburg, O.; Hammermann, J.; Lindner, M.; Stahl, M.; Muckenthaler, M.; Kohlmueller, D.; Happich, M.; Kulozik, A.E.; Stopsack, M.; Gahr, M.; et al. Five years of experience with biochemical cystic fibrosis newborn screening based on IRT/PAP in Germany. *Pediatr. Pulmonol.* **2015**, *50*, 655–664. [CrossRef] [PubMed]
16. Dankert-Roelse, J.E.; Bouva, M.J.; Jakobs, B.S.; Janssens, H.M.; Groot, K.D.W.-D.; Schönbeck, Y.; Gille, J.J.; Gulmans, V.A.; Verschoof-Puite, R.K.; Schielen, P.; et al. Newborn blood spot screening for cystic fibrosis with a four-step screening strategy in the Netherlands. *J. Cyst. Fibros.* **2019**, *18*, 54–63. [CrossRef] [PubMed]
17. Marcão, A.; Barreto, C.; Pereira, J.B.; Vaz, L.; Cavaco, J.; Casimiro, A.; Félix, M.; Silva, T.R.; Barbosa, T.; Freitas, C.; et al. Cystic Fibrosis Newborn Screening in Portugal: PAP Value in Populations with Stringent Rules for Genetic Studies. *Int. J. Neonatal Screen.* **2018**, *4*, 22. [CrossRef]
18. Sommerburg, O.; Krulišová, V.; Hammermann, J.; Lindner, M.; Stahl, M.; Muckenthaler, M.; Kohlmueller, D.; Happich, M.; Kulozik, A.E.; Votava, F.; et al. Comparison of different IRT-PAP protocols to screen newborns for cystic fibrosis in three central European populations. *J. Cyst. Fibros.* **2014**, *13*, 15–23. [CrossRef]
19. Castellani, C.; Duff, A.; Bell, S.C.; Heijerman, H.G.; Munck, A.; Ratjen, F.; Sermet-Gaudelus, I.; Southern, K.W.; Barben, J.; A Flume, P.; et al. ECFS best practice guidelines: The 2018 revision. *J. Cyst. Fibros.* **2018**, *17*, 153–178. [CrossRef]
20. Calvin, J.; Hogg, S.L.; McShane, D.; McAuley, S.A.; Iles, R.; Ross-Russell, R.; MacLean, F.M.; Heeley, M.E.; Heeley, A.F. Thirty-years of screening for cystic fibrosis in East Anglia. *Arch. Dis. Child.* **2012**, *97*, 1043–1047. [CrossRef]
21. Kharrazi, M.; Yang, J.; Bishop, T.; Lessing, S.; Young, S.; Graham, S.; Pearl, M.; Chow, H.; Ho, T.; Currier, R.; et al. Newborn Screening for Cystic Fibrosis in California. *Pediatrics* **2015**, *136*, 1062–1072. [CrossRef] [PubMed]
22. Sontag, M.; Lee, R.; Wright, D.; Freedenberg, D.; Sagel, S.D. Improving the Sensitivity and Positive Predictive Value in a Cystic Fibrosis Newborn Screening Program Using a Repeat Immunoreactive Trypsinogen and Genetic Analysis. *J. Pediatr.* **2016**, *175*, 150–158.e1. [CrossRef] [PubMed]
23. Lundman, E.; Gaup, H.J.; Bakkeheim, E.; Olafsdottir, E.J.; Rootwelt, T.; Storrøsten, O.T.; Pettersen, R.D. Implementation of newborn screening for cystic fibrosis in Norway. Results from the first three years. *J. Cyst. Fibros.* **2016**, *15*, 318–324. [CrossRef] [PubMed]
24. Skov, M.; Baekvad-Hansen, M.; Hougaard, D.M.; Skogstrand, K.; Lund, A.M.; Pressler, T.; Olesen, H.V.; Duno, M. Cystic fibrosis newborn screening in Denmark: Experience from the first 2 years. *Pediatr. Pulmonol.* **2019**, *55*, 549–555. [CrossRef]
25. Gemeinsamer Bundesausschuss. Kinder-Richtlinie: Änderung des Beschlusses zur Neufassung—Screening auf Mukoviszidose (Zystische Fibrose)—Tragende Gründe zum Beschluss. Available online: https://www.g-ba.de/informationen/beschluesse/2316/ (accessed on 3 November 2015).

26. Sommerburg, O.; Stahl, M.; Hammermann, J.; Okun, J.G.; Kulozik, A.; Hoffmann, G.; Mall, M. Neugeborenenscreening auf Mukoviszidose in Deutschland: Vergleich des neuen Screening-Protokolls mit einem Alternativprotokoll. *Klin. Pädiatrie* **2017**, *229*, 59–66. [CrossRef] [PubMed]
27. Zeyda, M.; (Medical University of Vienna, Vienna, Austria). Personal communication, 2020.
28. Gartner, S.; (Tilburg School of Catholic Theology, Tilburg, The Netherlands). Personal communication, 2020.

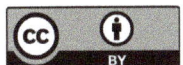

© 2020 by the authors. Licensee MDPI, Basel, Switzerland. This article is an open access article distributed under the terms and conditions of the Creative Commons Attribution (CC BY) license (http://creativecommons.org/licenses/by/4.0/).

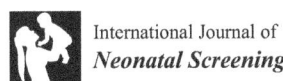 International Journal of
Neonatal Screening

Review

The Role of Extended *CFTR* Gene Sequencing in Newborn Screening for Cystic Fibrosis

Anne Bergougnoux [1], Maureen Lopez [2] and Emmanuelle Girodon [2,*]

[1] Molecular Genetics Laboratory, CHU Montpellier, EA7402 University of Montpellier, 34093 Montpellier CEDEX 5, France; anne.bergougnoux@inserm.fr
[2] Molecular Genetics Laboratory, Cochin Hospital, APHP. Centre, University of Paris, 75014 Paris, France; maureen.lopez@aphp.fr
* Correspondence: emmanuelle.girodon@aphp.fr; Tel.: +33-(0)158411924

Received: 25 February 2020; Accepted: 19 March 2020; Published: 21 March 2020

Abstract: There has been considerable progress in the implementation of newborn screening (NBS) programs for cystic fibrosis (CF), with DNA analysis being part of an increasing number of strategies. Thanks to advances in genomic sequencing technologies, *CFTR*-extended genetic analysis (EGA) by sequencing its coding regions has become affordable and has already been included as part of a limited number of core NBS programs, to the benefit of admixed populations. Based on results analysis of existing programs, the values and challenges of EGA are reviewed in the perspective of its implementation on a larger scale. Sensitivity would be increased at best by using EGA as a second tier, but this could be at the expense of positive predictive value, which improves, however, if EGA is applied after testing a variant panel. The increased detection of babies with an inconclusive diagnosis has proved to be a major drawback in programs using EGA. The lack of knowledge on pathogenicity and penetrance associated with numerous variants hinders the introduction of EGA as a second tier, but EGA with filtering for all known CF variants with full penetrance could be a solution. The issue of incomplete knowledge is a real challenge in terms of the implementation of NBS extended to many genetic diseases.

Keywords: cystic fibrosis; newborn screening; DNA analysis; next generation sequencing; extended genetic analysis

1. Introduction

For more than 40 years, newborn screening (NBS) programs for cystic fibrosis (CF) have been implemented across the world in Caucasian populations as pilot, regional, or national programs [1–6]. While early *CFTR* gene analysis is a key tool for the diagnosis of CF, for adapted follow-up, mutation-guided therapy, and genetic counseling, its place and extent in a core NBS program has long been a matter of debate. At present, there are a variety of established NBS programs [1], all starting with immunoreactive trypsinogen (IRT) measurement. DNA analysis is part of the majority of programs, most often performed in the second tier on the same dried blood spot as IRT measurement, and principally with search for a limited number of frequent variants. Some programs include extended *CFTR* gene analysis with next generation sequencing (NGS) focused on coding regions (referred to as extended genetic analysis (EGA)), mainly because of heterogeneous populations where the distribution and the frequency of CF-causing variants vary. These programs, however, lead to the detection of a high number of inconclusive cases, also referred to as Cystic Fibrosis Screen Positive, Inconclusive Diagnosis (CFSPID) in Europe or CFTR-related metabolic syndrome (CRMS) in the US, compared to the number of CF cases [1,7]. The definition of CRMS/CFSPID includes infants with a sweat chloride value between 30–59 mmol/L and zero or one CF-causing variant, or a sweat chloride value below 30 mmol/L and two *CFTR* variants, at least one of which has unclear phenotypic consequences [8,9].

Int. J. Neonatal Screen. **2020**, *6*, 23

Beyond technical and medical aspects, the choice of a NBS strategy is driven by the mutation spectrum in the screened population, the laboratory facilities, the health care system, the legal and economic aspects, and the acceptability by the population [10–13]. There is thus no universal model of NBS strategy. Nevertheless, there are minimal recommendations which have been issued by the European Society of Cystic Fibrosis (ECFS) [14], including, as performance criteria, a minimal positive predictive value (PPV) of 30% and a minimal diagnostic sensitivity of 95%. It is also an objective to minimize as much as possible the number of inconclusive cases and carrier detection. In the present article, we review the variety of NBS programs set up that include DNA analysis, along with their performance. The value, challenges, and drawbacks of *CFTR* EGA are then discussed, and then future prospects are eventually considered—in particular, in the view of a shift toward an extended NBS of a set of hereditary diseases by wide genomic analysis.

2. Overview of Newborn Screening Programs

A review of the literature was conducted to identify current NBS programs for CF and to update performance data, notably from the important review across Europe [1]. It is, however, possible that strategies have changed since the last available data. Where data were old and not detailed, they were not included in Table 1. In Europe, 22 countries have implemented NBS programs, 20 as national and two as regional programs. Fifteen programs use DNA analysis, mostly as a second tier after IRT measurement. Twelve countries use a variant panel only, and three have implemented EGA (Figure 1a). In North America, all Canada provinces follow an IRT/DNA panel strategy, as do the great majority of US states [5,6] (Figure 1b). Only six US states do not use DNA analysis in their core program. The states of California, Hawaii, and, recently, New York, which are composed of multi-ethnic and/or non-white populations, have introduced EGA as a third tier after analysis of a variant panel [5,7] (Personal Communication [15]). In Central and South America, some programs have been implemented, e.g., since 2001 in Brazil [16], but few have introduced DNA analysis in their strategy [17] (Figure 1c). In Australia and New Zealand, where NBS was implemented in 1989 and 1986, respectively, DNA analysis using mutation panels is now part of the strategy in the second tier [18,19] (Figure 1d).

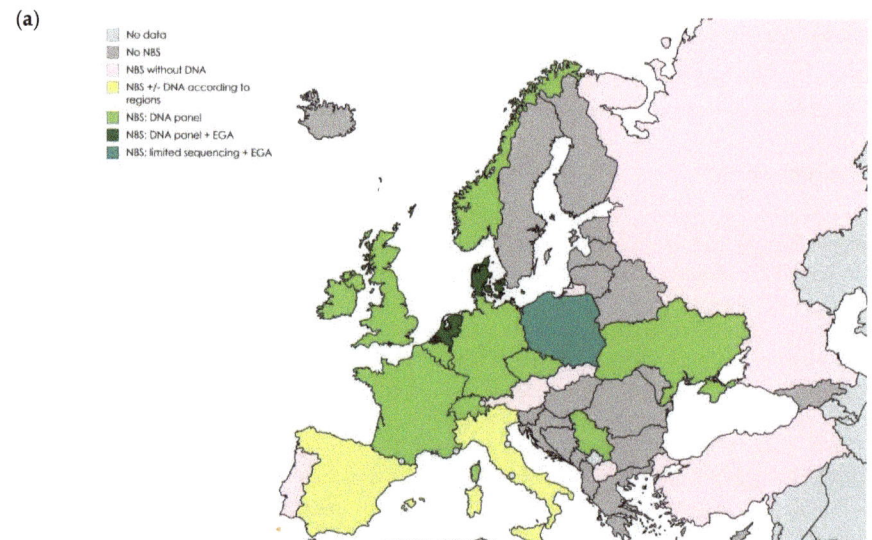

Figure 1. *Cont.*

(b)

(c)

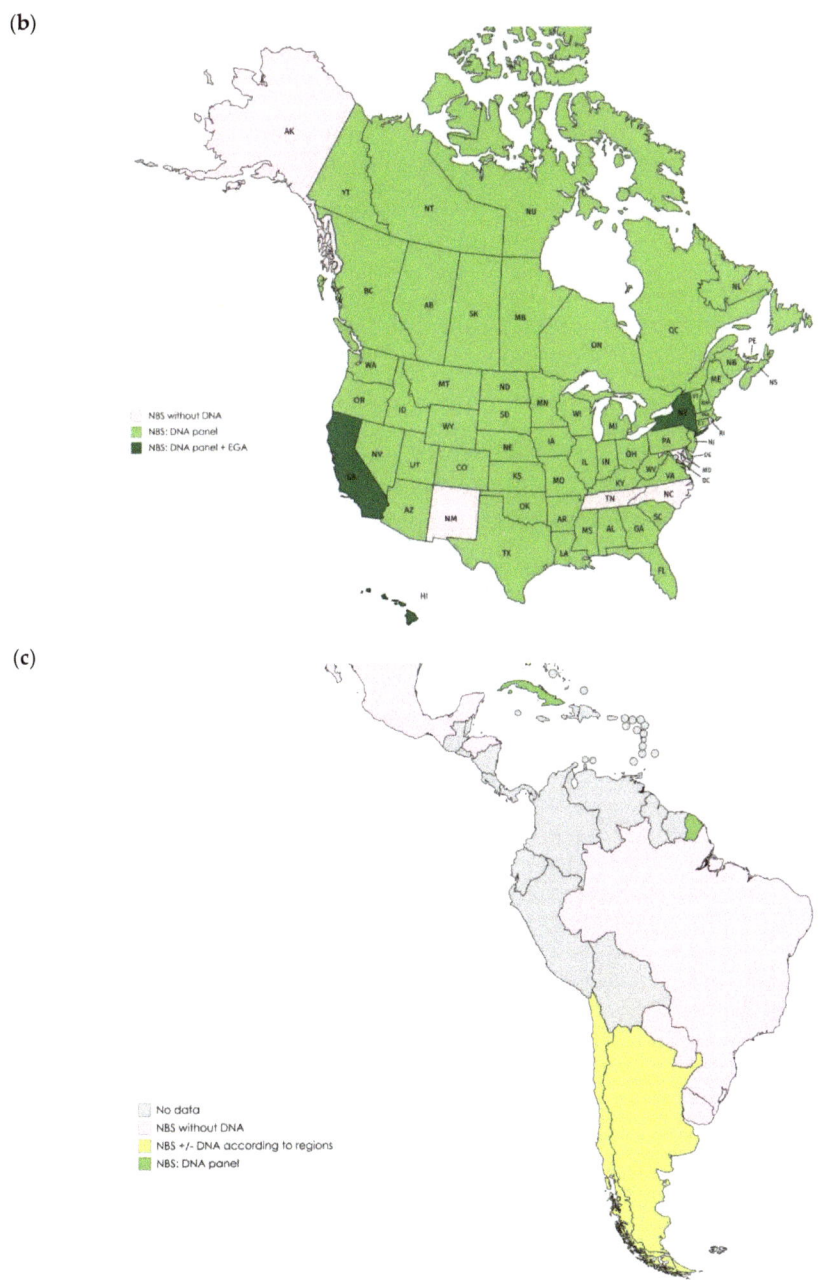

Figure 1. *Cont.*

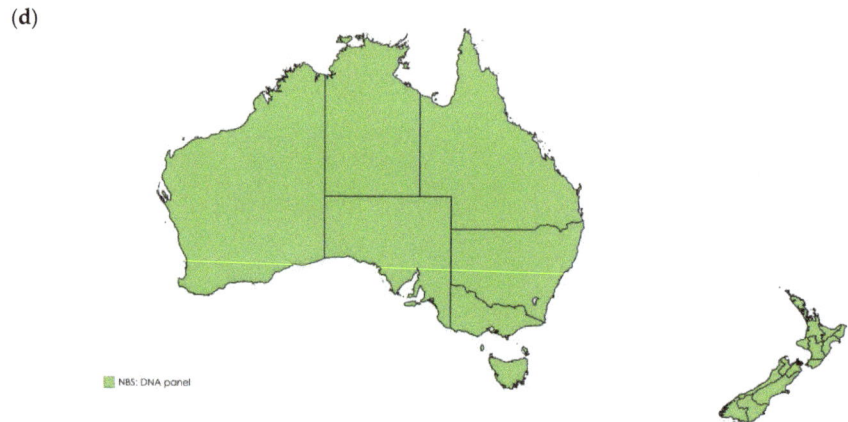

Figure 1. (**a**) In Europe, (**b**) in North America, (**c**) in South America, (**d**) in Australia and New Zealand. Newborn screening programs for cystic fibrosis (CF) according to the place of DNA analysis. NBS, newborn screening; EGA, extended *CFTR* genetic analysis.

Numerous programs have included a safety net protocol with the aim to identify CF infants who would be missed by testing variant panels because they carry two rare variants. Depending on the program, neonates with no variant but ultra-high IRT undergo either a second IRT measurement at 14–21 days or a direct sweat testing. In Denmark and the Netherlands, the safety net protocol leads to performing EGA. Safety net protocols lead to limiting false negatives cases, hence increasing the sensitivity of NBS programs, which is particularly effective in ethnic minority communities.

Comparing performances between different strategies using DNA analysis is a difficult task because of the considerable variability of protocols (Table 1), the changes over time in a country, the number of years since implementation, the duration of follow-up, the strategies and sensitivity of DNA analysis, and the monitoring of performance. Even when equivalent strategies are applied, there is variability in each step of the protocol, such as in the choice of the IRT cut-off value, the number of frequent variants screened by the panel, the use of a third or even fourth tier to minimize the number of children referred for sweat testing, or the safety net protocol (Table 1).

It is recommended to screen all pathogenic variants found at an incidence of 0.5% or higher according to geographical origins, or all variants accounting for more than 80% of CF alleles in the screened population [20]. The number of tested variants in NBS programs varies from 1 (F508del in Denmark and some states of the US [5,21]) to 388 (in New York State) (Personal Communication [15]).

Table 1. Strategies and performance of newborn screening programs for CF.

Countries/States	1st Tier	2nd Tier	3rd Tier	4th Tier	Safety Net	IRT1 > Cut Off	Sensitivity (wo MI)	PPV CF	Ratio CF:CFSPID	Carrier Frequency
Brazil (Sao Paulo) [16]										
Russia [22]										
Slovakia [1]		IRT				0.73–1.67%	86–100%	3–19%	ND 1.1:1 (Turkey)	NA
Turkey [23]										
Spain (Andalusia) [24]										
Austria [25]					IRT	0.97%		23%	25:1 *	NA
Portugal [26]		PAP				0.70%	94.4%	41%	ND	NA
Germany [27,28]		PAP	DNA (31)		ST	0.73%	96%	20%	5:1	1/44
US (Colorado, Texas, Wyoming) [29]		IRT	DNA (41–48)		ST	2.10%	96%	20%	10.8:1	1/13
US (Wisconsin) [30]	IRT	DNA (25)				ND	95%	9%	5.2:1	1/9.5
Australia (Victoria) [18]		DNA (12)				ND	96%	18.3%	7.8:1	ND
New Zealand [19]		DNA (3)				ND	100%	23%	ND	ND
Italy (Tuscany) [31]		DNA (66)				0.85%	89.5%	19.4%	2.85:1	1/16
France [32]		DNA (29)			IRT	0.50%	95%	34%	9:1	1/16
Switzerland [33]		DNA (7)			IRT	0.78%	97%	36%	17:1 *	1/11 *
Czech Republic [1,34]		DNA (50)			IRT	0.90%	94%	15%	7.5:1 *	1/21
Norway [35]		DNA (72)	DNA (20)		ST	0.8%	95%	43%	1:1	1/10
UK [1,36]		DNA (4)	DNA (29 or 31)	IRT	IRT	0.57% *	96%	76%	10.5:1 *	1/28 *
Denmark [21]		DNA (1)	EGA		EGA	3.70%	92%	85%	7:1	1/20
California [7]		DNA (40)	EGA			1.6%	92%	34%	0.65:1	1/25
Netherlands [37]		PAP	DNA (35)	EGA	EGA	0.98%	90%	63%	4:1	1/28
Poland [1,38]		DNA(limited seq)	EGA			0.6% *	100%	26%	1.2:1 *	1/15 *

CFSPID, CF screen positive, inconclusive diagnosis; DNA, refers to either variant panel analysis, with the number of variants screened indicated in brackets, or to limited CFTR gene sequencing (limited seq) in Poland; EGA, extended CFTR genetic analysis; IRT, immunoreactive trypsinogen; NA, not applicable; ND, not documented; ST, sweat test; PAP, pancreatitis-associated peptide; PPV, positive predictive value; wo MI, without meconium ileus. * Figures taken from [1]. Since the sensitivity of the panels used were not always available, they were not indicated in the table.

2.1. Programs Including Variant Panels Only

Most of the NBS protocols use a panel of frequent CF-causing variants after the first raised IRT value. Only Serbia, Ukraine, and some US states have included a second IRT measurement on a new blood sample before testing the panel, and Germany has included pancreatitis-associated peptide (PAP) measurement as a second tier before DNA analysis. The UK and Norway use a second DNA panel in neonates found to carry a variant of the first panel.

In most of these programs testing for a variant panel, infants carrying only one identified variant are referred for sweat testing in order to distinguish affected infants from healthy carriers. In the UK and Luxembourg, a second IRT measurement on a new sample is performed to select neonates found to carry one variant who will undergo sweat testing.

Inclusion into NBS programs of DNA analysis using variant panels appears to be at the benefice of both sensitivity and PPV compared to IRT/IRT protocols [1,11], with fewer false positive infants referred for sweat testing. However, despite the use of panels adapted to each population to achieve an optimal mutation detection rate, there remains disparity regarding sensitivity of the programs, with the majority above 95% (10/12 countries) according to ECFS recommendations [14]. Moreover, PPV varies from 3% to 76%. Of the 14 available PPV data sets, only four are above the ECFS target of 30%. Norway and the UK use DNA analysis in two successive panels, and the UK has also included a second IRT measurement after DNA analysis to select infants who will undergo sweat testing, which has raised the PPV up to 76%.

The CF:CFSPID ratio also varies between countries that use a DNA panel strategy, from 17:1 in Switzerland to 1:1 in Norway, along with the carrier frequency, from 1/9.5 in Wisconsin to 1/44 in Germany. This could be explained by different mutation detection rates of variant panels, implementation of a safety net protocol, IRT cut-off, and the frequency of carriers in each population. Indeed, the number of healthy carriers detected increases with the mutation detection rate [11].

2.2. Programs Including EGA

Six programs have implemented EGA in their strategy, applied after a first step of DNA analysis when one CF-causing variant is found. Denmark tests a single variant [21], the Netherlands a panel of 35 [37], California State tests a panel of 40 [7], Hawaii State a panel of 97 [5] and New York State a panel of 388 (Personal Communication [15]). Poland applies *CFTR* sequencing in two tiers: analysis of *CFTR* regions covering 77% of Polish variants, then all *CFTR* coding regions (Personal communication [39]). There is no available data on the performance of the programs in Hawaii State and in New York State where the strategy recently changed. While PPV in the Polish program is 26%, it is above 30% in the others, varying from 34% to 85% (Table 1). By contrast, the sensitivity displayed in the Polish program is 100%, compared with 90–92% for the other three.

Denmark have chosen a low IRT cut-off (50 ng/mL) and test for F508del which is carried by approximatively 96% of the CF patients on at least one allele [21]. F508del would be carried by only 79% of the CF patients in Poland on at least one allele, according to the 54.5% F508del allelic frequency among CF alleles [40]. The high frequency of F508del allele in Danish CF patients may also explain the better CF:CFSPID ratio in Denmark (7:1), compared with the ratio in California (0.65:1). The CF:CFSPID ratio of 4:1 in the Netherlands is probably due to the additional step of PAP measurement that minimizes the number of positive screened newborns.

The rate of CF carriers detected through NBS also varies, from 1/15 in Poland to 1/28 in the Netherlands.

3. Values and Challenges of *CFTR* Extended Genetic Analysis

Assessing the value of EGA in NBS strategies is not a simple matter, given the few experiences documented, the different protocols followed, and the variable number of years since implementation. The analysis and the discussion below take into account these experiences, as well as considerations beyond to assess the value and challenges of EGA, either as a third-tier step after testing for a variant panel or directly as a second-tier step. They are summarized in Table 2.

Table 2. Strengths and weaknesses of extended *CFTR* gene analysis in newborn screening programs for CF, as a second- or third-tier step (IRT/EGA or IRT/DNA panel/EGA), compared to strategies including tests for variant panels only (IRT/DNA panel).

Strengths	Weaknesses
High PPV	but ...
• Reduction of false positive results of NBS strategy with EGA in the third tier, hence: • Reduction of unnecessary sweat tests with EGA in the third tier	• Low CF:CFSPID ratio, expected to be further lowered if using EGA in the second tier because of: • Numerous babies with two *CFTR* VUS or VVCC with EGA in the second tier, leading to unnecessary sweat tests, thus at the expense of PPV • The important need for follow-up of infants with CRMS/CFSPID
High Sensitivity	but ...
• Highest expected sensitivity with EGA in the second tier • Best equity between populations, adapted for minorities carrying rare variants • Unmasking new couples at risk of having a CF child (carrier detection)	• Misdiagnosis of CF or CRMS/CFSPID if referring to CFTR2 only • Increased number of carriers detected, including carriers of VUS and VVCC, especially with EGA in the second tier
Technically feasible	but ... requires optimal healthcare system organization
• NGS already in routine in laboratories for several years • Coverage of all known and unknown variants	• NBS sequencing platform development or reorganization, especially if EGA in the second tier • Questionable cost-effectiveness of the NBS program because of its impacts beyond • Technical limitations (homopolymers, large deletions, deep intronic variants) depending on the technique and the design
Increased knowledge on *CFTR* variants	but ... raises questions on variant interpretation
• Database enrichment and genotype–phenotype studies • Genetic counseling for future cases/pregnancies	• Increased number of VUS • Need for additional in vitro/ex vivo experiments and clinical examinations for variant interpretation • Disease penetrance unknown for many variants
More precise medical care	but ... raises ethical questions
• Detection of the two disease-causing variants in a single step • Earlier access to treatment	• Possible delay at the first medical visit according to ECFS recommendations [14] • Psychological impact of long-term follow up of infants with CRMS/CFSPID • Detection of patients who may not be symptomatic before adulthood and are at an unknown risk of developing a CFTR-related disorder

CFSPID, CF screen positive, inconclusive diagnosis; CRMS, CFTR-related metabolic syndrome; EGA, extended *CFTR* genetic analysis; IRT, immunoreactive trypsinogen; NBS, newborn screening; NGS, Next Generation Sequencing; VVCC, variant of varying clinical consequence; VUS, variant of uncertain or unknown significance.

3.1. Values of CFTR Extended Genetic Analysis in Newborn Screening Programs for CF

3.1.1. Reduction of NBS False-Positive Results and Improvement of the PPV

Inclusion of EGA as a third tier after testing a variant panel appears to reduce the number of NBS false-positive results, thus the consecutive number of unnecessary sweat tests, and to improve the PPV as compared to programs that include testing for variant panels only (Table 1) [41]. Sweat chloride measurement, a key component for confirmation of CF, indeed requires a specific local CF center organization with a dedicated laboratory, as well as strong experience and routine practice of physicians for optimal performance and high quality [42,43].

3.1.2. Best Equity of CF Screening between Populations

One of the main rationales and benefits of implementation of EGA in NBS programs for CF is better equity for multi-ethnic communities compared to variant panels [43]. Even if a unique panel has been initially designed to cover the most frequent CF variants of the local population, migration flows modifying the ethnic mix would require recurrent updates to maintain high sensitivity of the test. Any DNA panel, even of large size, will miss rare variants.

3.1.3. Increased Knowledge of the Phenotypical Spectrum of CFTR Variants

EGA also opens the opportunity to enrich our knowledge on the phenotypical spectrum and penetrance associated with *CFTR* variants, especially variants of varying clinical consequences (VVCC) and variants of unknown significance (VUS). Long term follow-up of patients who carry a VUS in *trans* of a CF-causing variant would help define variant pathogenicity and enrich locus-specific databases (CFMDB [44], CFTR2, [45], and *CFTR*-France, [46]).

3.1.4. Earlier Diagnosis and Access to Treatment

In the era of precision medicine, extended sequencing of the *CFTR* gene in IRT-positive neonates would detect all actionable variants for which efficient modulators of CFTR protein are now available. An early molecular diagnosis for CF would thus ensure early access to treatment. Comparison of the delay at the first medical visit may not seem better in programs that include EGA, but the delay until the two CF-causing variants are detected would be much shorter.

3.2. Challenges

3.2.1. Healthcare System Organization

Implementation of EGA in NBS programs for CF raises major challenges. Not only should the costs of the core strategy, which may vary considerably [7,13,47], be taken into consideration but so should those incurred by sweat testing if EGA is performed in the second tier, variant functional testing, genetic investigations in the parents, medical visits, and long-term follow-up of all screen-positive infants, either diagnosed with CF or with an inconclusive diagnosis.

3.2.2. Technical Issues

NBS Sequencing Platforms Development or Reorganization

Sequencing for NBS can be done on the same platform as for routine diagnosis already in place in laboratories. However, NBS requires a specific organization with optimized preanalytical protocols on dried-drop specimen and a specialized molecular genetics team for *CFTR* variant interpretation. Moreover, priority has to be given to the NBS process in order to respect ECFS recommendations about the timeliness of results.

Interestingly, the molecular strategy applied in the states of California and New York includes a single technical assay for DNA analysis, that is, NGS sequencing of all *CFTR* exons and recurrent deep intronic variants, with a two-step bioinformatic analysis: an initial, predefined variant panel is run simultaneously to a deep scan that is masked, and the mask is lifted if only one CF-causing variant is detected. This unique molecular strategy may further improve the timeliness of results as compared to other approaches.

Sequencing and Bioinformatics Limitations for Variant Detection

Technical limitations include sequencing errors in homopolymer-rich sequences or in pseudo-homologous genomic regions [48] and the risk of missing short insertions or deletions because of misalignment of sequence reads. It is thus recommended to use several variant callers in the NGS pipeline in order to maximize variant detection efficiency [49], and this should be considered in the evaluation of costs. Inappropriate or insufficient design coverage could lead to missing large deletions or insertions and variants located in deep intronic regions. The design should thus be adapted and continuously updated accordingly [50,51]. Low DNA quality and quantity extracted of dried-blot samples are other constraints for the detection of large deletions and insertions [52].

Positive results should be confirmed by an independent assay on a second DNA dilution for identity monitoring, as in other programs. Using EGA, a higher number of variants is expected to require confirmation because of an increased detection and the possible technical limitation of NGS. Familial segregation analysis is also essential to confirm compound heterozygosity and to avoid false-positive results due to numerous complex alleles reported in the *CFTR* gene [46,53,54]. Parents' blood sampling for DNA analysis should therefore be carried out optimally during the first visit so that medical care is not delayed. These essential experiments, whose numbers will inevitably increase with EGA being included in NBS, especially as a second-tier step, have to be considered for medico-economic studies.

3.2.3. Byproducts of NBS for CF and Ethical Issues

Increased Detection of Inconclusive Diagnosis

The identification of a substantial number of VUS or VVCC in neonates without any clinical symptoms and leading to an inconclusive diagnosis is a major drawback observed in the few experiences of EGA in NBS. In strategies that include EGA as a core component, neonates found to carry two variants (one of which being a VUS) and to have a negative sweat test fall into the category of inconclusive diagnosis, while in other strategies that include variant panels only, these neonates would be classified as healthy carriers. Indeed, since the sweat test is negative, DNA analysis stops at the step of variant panel and the VUS will not be identified. Implementation of EGA as a second-tier analysis after a raised IRT would lead to the further detection of infants with an inconclusive diagnosis who would have a negative sweat test and carry other kinds of genotypes, composed of two VVCC, a VVCC and a VUS, or two VUS.

Despite accumulation of considerable data on *CFTR* variants in locus-specific variant databases (CFMDB, CFTR2, *CFTR*-France), epidemiological data and genotype–phenotype correlations still miss most rare genetic *CFTR* variants, which are sometimes restricted to one family. Furthermore, the number of new variants is steadily increasing, as illustrated in the California program, where 78 out of 303 rare variants were novel [7]. On the other hand, databases may provide discordant information that one should be aware of, notably because of their different designs. Data in CFTR2 are provided from national registries of CF patients and thus represent the "tip of the iceberg" of all possible phenotypes associated with a given genotype. By contrast, *CFTR*-France collects genetic and clinical data from patients with CF and CFTR-RD and from asymptomatic individuals, and so some variants are differently classified in the two databases. In addition, variants that are not referred to in the list of 432 described in CFTR2 have been classified as VUS in several programs [7,55,56], despite their description in the literature and other databases, either as CF-causing or as non-CF-causing. As a consequence, the number of CRMS/CFSPID observed in programs that include EGA may be overestimated and the ratio of CF:CFSPID artificially biased.

The risk that neonates with an inconclusive diagnosis will develop symptoms consistent with CF, even in a less typical form, with a possible delayed positive conversion of the sweat test [57,58] is still unknown. Nevertheless, parents should be informed on the longer-term risks that their child may develop clinical symptoms of CF. Ex vivo electrophysiological explorations on nasal epithelium, organoids, or rectal biopsies and in vitro experiments on heterologous immortalized cell systems reproducing DNA changes may help interpret variant pathogenicity and better evaluate the risk of developing clinical CF. A follow-up longer than two years is then critical [56,58]. However, the full penetrance associated with some VVCC may not be apparent until adulthood [55]. One may wonder whether the detection of patients who will not be symptomatic before adulthood is desirable. The frequency of variants and genotypes in the general population should be considered to evaluate the risk of a particular genotype to cause clinical CF; in other words, the penetrance of clinical CF in individuals carrying a given genotype. This was previously shown to be very low for R117H [59], an observation which led to its withdrawal from NBS variant panels [27,32], and, more recently, for the T5 variants and other variants commonly identified in inconclusive cases [60]. Such epidemiological data emphasize the importance of documenting the penetrance of variants before widely implementing EGA in core NBS programs.

The increased detection of inconclusive cases when using EGA strategies should thus be anticipated with regard to the organization of CF centers, the costs of follow-up, and the additional investigations for variant interpretation. Moreover, additional studies on psychological consequences [61] of the long-term follow-up of these patients are needed before implementation of EGA as a global model.

Carrier Detection and Genetic Counseling

Detection of healthy carriers, heterozygous for one CF-causing variant, is another unwanted result of NBS, though it has been considered a benefit that enables reproductive planning [62]. It will inevitably be increased by a more extensive DNA analysis in NBS strategy [10] and will have a cost for increased referrals in the families. Indeed, once a CF-causing variant is detected, a "cascade" genetic screening is recommended in relatives [63,64].

Here, again, as for inconclusive cases uncertainty about VUS and VVCC is puzzling and complicates genetic counseling. It is thus not only the higher number of healthy carriers of known CF-causing variants that healthcare professionals have to deal with, but the even higher expected number of carriers of VVCC and VUS. Updated information should be provided to families as knowledge evolves on variant pathogenicity, but such recalls could also generate anxiety. Population genetics data should not be neglected, as it has been shown that a number of variants classified as VUS or VVCC in CFTR2 actually have a frequency in the general population that argues against a severe impact, as for c.2620-26A>G, R74W, R117H, I556V, or D1270N [65]. The risk is to consider neonates as carriers of a CF-causing variant and to offer inappropriate genetic counseling and testing in the family, and eventually inappropriate prenatal diagnosis. In view of the expanding strategies that include EGA, guidelines should be issued on these matters to minimize as much as possible these byproducts.

4. Conclusions and Perspectives

Considerable expansion has been observed in the implementation of NBS programs for CF, with DNA analysis being part of an increasing number of strategies. While testing for *CFTR* gene variant panels as a second tier has been proven to improve the performance and reduce the false-positive rates, the value and place of *CFTR* EGA before the diagnostic step of sweat testing is still not obvious. The performance is indeed the result of all steps, starting with IRT cut-off values. Implementation of EGA in the NBS process, which has been greatly facilitated by advances in genomic sequencing technologies, is expected to achieve an optimal sensitivity in ethnically diverse populations and a faster genetic diagnosis in CF infants without the need of another sample. EGA has been implemented in three European countries and three US states only, with different mutational backgrounds and different protocols, so that comparison remains difficult. The major drawback of approaches that include EGA is the unwanted detection of neonates with an inconclusive diagnosis, with a CF:CFSPID ratio varying from one program to another, but which is as low as 1.2:1 in Poland [1] and 0.65:1 in California [7]. This challenging situation, leading to uncertainty for healthcare professionals and families, also generates costs that should be considered in the health economic evaluation of a program before its implementation. Based on data indicative of a low penetrance for a set of variants identified in inconclusive cases [59,60], it is likely that the detection of neonates carrying a true CF-causing variant in *trans* of such a variant would considerably increase in a program based on IRT/EGA, thus finally requiring a high number of sweat tests to be performed, not to mention other tests, follow-up visits, and parents' resulting anxiety. Therefore, the significant risk reported for neonates with an inconclusive diagnosis to develop a CF disease [58] might be considerably lowered as many more cases are detected through EGA before sweat testing. By contrast, removal of R117H from the variant panel of the French NBS program led to dramatically improved performance, with the PPV increasing from 16% to 34% and the ratio CF:CFSPID from 6.3:1 to 9:1 [32].

Eventually, based on technological advances in genomic sequencing and the reduction of costs along with the steadily increasing implementation of NBS programs in multi-ethnic populations or populations where common variants are not included in current DNA panels, an optimal compromise to improve performance and minimize side effects would be to perform EGA with bioinformatics targeting a wide panel of fully penetrant CF-causing variants, including large deletions and deep-intronic variants, as recently implemented in New York State. EGA without applying any bioinformatic filter or without any additional step as IRT or PAP to limit the number of infants subjected to sweat testing might be detrimental, as long as the clinical impact and penetrance data associated with variants are not well documented. In view of this, the collection of data on the extended follow-up of neonates detected with an inconclusive diagnosis is of the utmost importance [58].

The question of the role of EGA in the context of NBS does not only focus on CF. Whole exome sequencing and whole genome sequencing are nowadays affordable due to a significant reduction of costs. The relevance of implementing extended NBS for numerous genetic diseases is currently debated [66–68], which again raises the unsolved question of the interpretation of rare variants all along the genome. In this respect, comprehensive information on genetic issues should be given to the parents prior to NBS. Expanded preconception carrier screening for recessive disorders is also under consideration in countries following an overall positive attitude of the general population [69], depending on ethnical and geographical origin, degree of consanguinity, and type of disorders. Preconception CF carrier screening has already been implemented in the US, Israël, and Northeast Italy [70]. Such a health public policy aims to detect most at-risk couples and this ineluctably impacts on the timing for a CF diagnosis and on the prevalence of CF births [71], which would then raise the question of the relevance of NBS. Reproductive attitudes would also inevitably change, as recently underlined [72]. Requests for prenatal diagnoses may increase, especially where non-invasive procedures have been recently available [73,74], but where a diagnosis of CF is made, with the growing availability of mutation-guided therapy the option of the continuation of pregnancy could be preferred over termination.

In conclusion, designation of an optimal NBS program remains necessarily country-dependent. The introduction of EGA as a second tier without filtering of CF variants has major drawbacks that are yet unsolved and may negatively impact the organization of care and the cost-effectiveness of NBS for CF. Consideration of any change in strategy should be carefully evaluated, planned, and monitored. This reinforces the need to adopt a standardized approach to collect data to the benefice of performance comparison. Taking all of these elements into account will ensure the sustainability of implemented NBS programs.

Author Contributions: Conception and design of the study, A.B. and E.G.; review of literature data, writing of the manuscript, A.B., M.L. and E.G. All authors have read and agreed to the published version of the manuscript.

Funding: This work received no external funding.

Acknowledgments: The authors are grateful to Michele Caggana for recent data on the New York State program, Dorota Sands for data on the Poland program, and Carlo Castellani for valuable discussion.

Conflicts of Interest: The authors declare no conflicts of interest.

References

1. Barben, J.; Castellani, C.; Dankert-Roelse, J.; Gartner, S.; Kashirskaya, N.; Linnane, B.; Mayell, S.; Munck, A.; Sands, D.; Sommerburg, O.; et al. The expansion and performance of national newborn screening programmes for cystic fibrosis in Europe. *J. Cyst. Fibros.* **2017**, *16*, 207–213. [CrossRef] [PubMed]
2. NSWG Annual Report 2018. Available online: https://www.ecfs.eu/sites/default/files/general-content-files/working-groups/NSWG%20annual%20report%202018v2.pdf (accessed on 21 February 2020).
3. Massie, J.; Clements, B.; The Australian Paediatric Respiratory Group. Diagnosis of cystic fibrosis after newborn screening: The Australasian experience—twenty years and five million babies later: A consensus statement from the Australasian paediatric respiratory group. *Pediatr. Pulmonol.* **2005**, *39*, 440–446. [CrossRef] [PubMed]
4. Byrnes, C.A.; Vidmar, S.; Cheney, J.L.; Carlin, J.B.; Armstrong, D.S.; Cooper, P.J.; Grimwood, K.; Moodie, M.; Robertson, C.F.; Rosenfeld, M.; et al. Prospective evaluation of respiratory exacerbations in children with cystic fibrosis from newborn screening to 5 years of age. *Thorax* **2013**, *68*, 643–651. [CrossRef] [PubMed]
5. Pique, L.; Graham, S.; Pearl, M.; Kharrazi, M.; Schrijver, I. Cystic fibrosis newborn screening programs: Implications of the *CFTR* variant spectrum in nonwhite patients. *Genet. Med.* **2017**, *19*, 36–44. [CrossRef]
6. Mak, D.Y.F.; Sykes, J.; Stephenson, A.L.; Lands, L.C. The benefits of newborn screening for cystic fibrosis: The Canadian experience. *J. Cyst. Fibros.* **2016**, *15*, 302–308. [CrossRef]
7. Kharrazi, M.; Yang, J.; Bishop, T.; Lessing, S.; Young, S.; Graham, S.; Pearl, M.; Chow, H.; Ho, T.; Currier, R.; et al. Newborn Screening for Cystic Fibrosis in California. *Pediatrics* **2015**, *136*, 1062–1072. [CrossRef]
8. Farrell, P.M.; White, T.B.; Howenstine, M.S.; Munck, A.; Parad, R.B.; Rosenfeld, M.; Sommerburg, O.; Accurso, F.J.; Davies, J.C.; Rock, M.J.; et al. Diagnosis of Cystic Fibrosis in Screened Populations. *J. Pediatr.* **2017**, *181*, S33–S44. [CrossRef]
9. Southern, K.W.; Barben, J.; Gartner, S.; Munck, A.; Castellani, C.; Mayell, S.J.; Davies, J.C.; Winters, V.; Murphy, J.; Salinas, D.; et al. Inconclusive diagnosis after a positive newborn bloodspot screening result for cystic fibrosis; clarification of the harmonised international definition. *J. Cyst. Fibros.* **2019**, *18*, 778–780. [CrossRef]
10. Castellani, C.; Southern, K.W.; Brownlee, K.; Dankert Roelse, J.; Duff, A.; Farrell, M.; Mehta, A.; Munck, A.; Pollitt, R.; Sermet-Gaudelus, I.; et al. European best practice guidelines for cystic fibrosis neonatal screening. *J. Cyst. Fibros.* **2009**, *8*, 153–173. [CrossRef]
11. Castellani, C.; Massie, J.; Sontag, M.; Southern, K.W. Newborn screening for cystic fibrosis. *Lancet Respir. Med.* **2016**, *4*, 653–661. [CrossRef]
12. Castellani, C.; Linnane, B.; Pranke, I.; Cresta, F.; Sermet-Gaudelus, I.; Peckham, D. Cystic Fibrosis Diagnosis in Newborns, Children, and Adults. *Semin. Respir. Crit. Care Med.* **2019**, *40*, 701–714. [CrossRef] [PubMed]
13. Schmidt, M.; Werbrouck, A.; Verhaeghe, N.; de Wachter, E.; Simoens, S.; Annemans, L.; Putman, K. A model-based economic evaluation of four newborn screening strategies for cystic fibrosis in Flanders, Belgium. *Acta Clin. Belg.* **2019**, 1–9. [CrossRef] [PubMed]
14. Castellani, C.; Duff, A.J.A.; Bell, S.C.; Heijerman, H.G.M.; Munck, A.; Ratjen, F.; Sermet-Gaudelus, I.; Southern, K.W.; Barben, J.; Flume, P.A.; et al. ECFS best practice guidelines: The 2018 revision. *J. Cyst. Fibros.* **2018**, *17*, 153–178. [CrossRef] [PubMed]
15. Caggana, M. (New York State Department of Health, Albany, NY 12208, USA). Personal communication, 2020.
16. Rodrigues, R.; Magalhaes, P.K.R.; Fernandes, M.I.M.; Gabetta, C.S.; Ribeiro, A.F.; Pedro, K.P.; Valdetaro, F.; Santos, J.L.F.; de Souza, R.M.; Pazin Filho, A.; et al. Neonatal screening for cystic fibrosis in São Paulo State, Brazil: A pilot study. *Braz. J. Med. Biol. Res.* **2009**, *42*, 973–978. [CrossRef] [PubMed]
17. XI Congreso Latinoamericano de Errores Inatos del Metabolismo y Pesquisa Neonatal. 2019. Available online: http://www.sleimpn2019.org/index.php/trabajos/posters-pesquisa-neonatal (accessed on 21 February 2020).
18. Massie, R.J.H.; Curnow, L.; Glazner, J.; Armstrong, D.S.; Francis, I. Lessons learned from 20 years of newborn screening for cystic fibrosis. *Med. J. Aust.* **2012**, *196*, 67–70. [CrossRef]
19. Ministry of Health. *Newborn Metabolic Screening Programme: Annual Report 2017*; Ministry of Health: Wellington, New Zealand, 2018.

20. Ross, L.F. Newborn Screening for Cystic Fibrosis: A Lesson in Public Health Disparities. *J. Pediatr.* **2008**, *153*, 308–313. [CrossRef]
21. Skov, M.; Bækvad-Hansen, M.; Hougaard, D.M.; Skogstrand, K.; Lund, A.M.; Pressler, T.; Olesen, H.V.; Duno, M. Cystic fibrosis newborn screening in Denmark: Experience from the first 2 years. *Pediatr. Pulmonol.* **2020**, *55*, 549–555. [CrossRef]
22. Tolstova, V.D.; Kashirskaya, N.Y.; Kapranov, N.I.; Khodunova, A.A.; Denisenkova, E.V.; Smazhil, E.V. First results of newborn screening program for CF in Russia. *J. Cyst. Fibros.* **2008**, *7*, S13. [CrossRef]
23. Başaran, A.E.; Başaran, A.; Uygun, D.F.K.; Alper, Ö.; Acican, D.; BïNgöl, A. Initial regional evaluation of the Cystic Fibrosis Newborn Screening Program: Data from the Mediterranean coast of Turkey. *Turk. J. Med. Sci.* **2019**, *49*, 1655–1661.
24. Delgado Pecellín, I.; Pérez Ruiz, E.; Álvarez Ríos, A.I.; Delgado Pecellín, C.; Yahyaoui Macías, R.; Carrasco Hernández, L.; Marcos Luque, I.; Caro Aguilera, P.; Moreno Valera, M.J.; Quintana Gallego, M.E. Results of the Andalusian Cystic Fibrosis Neonatal Screening Program, 5 Years After Implementation. *Arch. Bronconeumol.* **2018**, *54*, 551–558. [CrossRef]
25. Renner, S.; Schanzer, A.; Metz, T.; Szépfalusi, Z.; Zeyda, M. CF newborn screening in Austria: After 20 years changing the algorithm from IRT/IRT to IRT/PAP/IRT. *J. Cyst. Fibros.* **2018**, *17*, S18. [CrossRef]
26. Marcão, A.; Barreto, C.; Pereira, L.; Vaz, L.; Cavaco, J.; Casimiro, A.; Félix, M.; Silva, T.; Barbosa, T.; Freitas, C.; et al. Cystic Fibrosis Newborn Screening in Portugal: PAP Value in Populations with Stringent Rules for Genetic Studies. *Int. J. Neonatal Screen.* **2018**, *4*, 22. [CrossRef]
27. Sommerburg, O.; Stahl, M.; Hammermann, J.; Okun, J.; Kulozik, A.; Hoffmann, G.; Mall, M. Neugeborenenscreening auf Mukoviszidose in Deutschland: Vergleich des neuen Screening-Protokolls mit einem Alternativprotokoll. *Klin. Padiatr.* **2017**, *229*, 59–66. [CrossRef] [PubMed]
28. Brockow, I.; Nennstiel, U. Parents' experience with positive newborn screening results for cystic fibrosis. *Eur. J. Pediatr.* **2019**, *178*, 803–809. [CrossRef]
29. Sontag, M.K.; Lee, R.; Wright, D.; Freedenberg, D.; Sagel, S.D. Improving the Sensitivity and Positive Predictive Value in a Cystic Fibrosis Newborn Screening Program Using a Repeat Immunoreactive Trypsinogen and Genetic Analysis. *J. Pediatr.* **2016**, *175*, 150–158. [CrossRef]
30. Rock, M.J.; Hoffman, G.; Laessig, R.H.; Kopish, G.J.; Litsheim, T.J.; Farrell, P.M. Newborn screening for cystic fibrosis in Wisconsin: Nine-year experience with routine trypsinogen/DNA testing. *J. Pediatr.* **2005**, *147*, S73–S77. [CrossRef]
31. Terlizzi, V.; Mergni, G.; Buzzetti, R.; Centrone, C.; Zavataro, L.; Braggion, C. Cystic fibrosis screen positive inconclusive diagnosis (CFSPID): Experience in Tuscany, Italy. *J. Cyst. Fibros.* **2019**, *18*, 484–490. [CrossRef]
32. Munck, A.; Delmas, D.; Audrézet, M.-P.; Lemonnier, L.; Cheillan, D.; Roussey, M. Optimization of the French cystic fibrosis newborn screening programme by a centralized tracking process. *J. Med. Screen.* **2018**, *25*, 6–12. [CrossRef]
33. Rueegg, C.S.; Kuehni, C.E.; Gallati, S.; Baumgartner, M.; Torresani, T.; Barben, J. One-Year Evaluation of a Neonatal Screening Program for Cystic Fibrosis in Switzerland. *Dtsch. Arztebl. Int.* **2013**, *110*, 356–363. [CrossRef]
34. Krulišová, V.; Balaščaková, M.; Skalická, V.; Piskáčková, T.; Holubová, A.; Paděrová, J.; Křenková, P.; Dvořáková, L.; Zemková, D.; Kračmar, P.; et al. Prospective and parallel assessments of cystic fibrosis newborn screening protocols in the Czech Republic: IRT/DNA/IRT versus IRT/PAP and IRT/PAP/DNA. *Eur. J. Pediatr.* **2012**, *171*, 1223–1229. [CrossRef]
35. Lundman, E.; Gaup, H.J.; Bakkeheim, E.; Olafsdottir, E.J.; Rootwelt, T.; Storrøsten, O.T.; Pettersen, R.D. Implementation of newborn screening for cystic fibrosis in Norway. Results from the first three years. *J. Cyst. Fibros.* **2016**, *15*, 318–324. [CrossRef] [PubMed]
36. Schlüter, D.K.; Southern, K.W.; Dryden, C.; Diggle, P.; Taylor-Robinson, D. Impact of newborn screening on outcomes and social inequalities in cystic fibrosis: A UK CF registry-based study. *Thorax* **2020**, *75*, 123–131. [CrossRef] [PubMed]
37. Dankert-Roelse, J.E.; Bouva, M.J.; Jakobs, B.S.; Janssens, H.M.; de Winter-de Groot, K.M.; Schönbeck, Y.; Gille, J.J.P.; Gulmans, V.A.M.; Verschoof-Puite, R.K.; Schielen, P.C.J.I.; et al. Newborn blood spot screening for cystic fibrosis with a four-step screening strategy in the Netherlands. *J. Cyst. Fibros.* **2019**, *18*, 54–63. [CrossRef] [PubMed]

38. Sands, D.; Zybert, K.; Mierzejewska, E.; Oltarzewski, M. Diagnosing cystic fibrosis in newborn screening in Poland—15 years of experience. *Dev. Period Med.* **2015**, *19*, 16–24.
39. Sands, D. (Zaklad Mukowiscydozy, Instytut Matki i Dziecka, Kasprzaka 17a, 01-211 Warsow, Poland). Personal communication, 2020.
40. Ziętkiewicz, E.; Rutkiewicz, E.; Pogorzelski, A.; Klimek, B.; Voelkel, K.; Witt, M. *CFTR* mutations spectrum and the efficiency of molecular diagnostics in Polish cystic fibrosis patients. *PLoS ONE* **2014**, *9*, e89094. [CrossRef]
41. Currier, R.J.; Sciortino, S.; Liu, R.; Bishop, T.; Alikhani Koupaei, R.; Feuchtbaum, L. Genomic sequencing in cystic fibrosis newborn screening: What works best, two-tier predefined *CFTR* mutation panels or second-tier *CFTR* panel followed by third-tier sequencing? *Genet. Med.* **2017**, *19*, 1159–1163. [CrossRef]
42. Cirilli, N.; Southern, K.W.; Buzzetti, R.; Barben, J.; Nährlich, L.; Munck, A.; Wilschanski, M.; De Boeck, K.; Derichs, N. Real life practice of sweat testing in Europe. *J. Cyst. Fibros.* **2018**, *17*, 325–332. [CrossRef]
43. Schrijver, I.; Pique, L.; Graham, S.; Pearl, M.; Cherry, A.; Kharrazi, M. The Spectrum of *CFTR* Variants in Nonwhite Cystic Fibrosis Patients: Implications for Molecular Diagnostic Testing. *J. Mol. Diagn.* **2016**, *18*, 39–50. [CrossRef]
44. Cystic Fibrosis Mutation Data Base (CFMDB). Available online: http://www.genet.sickkids.on.ca/ (accessed on 21 February 2020).
45. Sosnay, P.R.; Siklosi, K.R.; Van Goor, F.; Kaniecki, K.; Yu, H.; Sharma, N.; Ramalho, A.S.; Amaral, M.D.; Dorfman, R.; Zielenski, J.; et al. Defining the disease liability of variants in the cystic fibrosis transmembrane conductance regulator gene. *Nat. Genet.* **2013**, *45*, 1160–1167. [CrossRef]
46. Claustres, M.; Thèze, C.; des Georges, M.; Baux, D.; Girodon, E.; Bienvenu, T.; Audrezet, M.-P.; Dugueperoux, I.; Férec, C.; Lalau, G.; et al. *CFTR*-France, a national relational patient database for sharing genetic and phenotypic data associated with rare *CFTR* variants. *Hum. Mutat.* **2017**, *38*, 1297–1315. [CrossRef]
47. Wells, J.; Rosenberg, M.; Hoffman, G.; Anstead, M.; Farrell, P.M. A Decision-Tree Approach to Cost Comparison of Newborn Screening Strategies for Cystic Fibrosis. *Pediatrics* **2012**, *129*, e339–e347. [CrossRef] [PubMed]
48. Deeb, K.K.; Metcalf, J.D.; Sesock, K.M.; Shen, J.; Wensel, C.A.; Rippel, L.I.; Smith, M.; Chapman, M.S.; Zhang, S. The c.1364C>A (p.A455E) Mutation in the *CFTR* Pseudogene Results in an Incorrectly Assigned Carrier Status by a Commonly Used Screening Platform. *J. Mol. Diagn.* **2015**, *17*, 360–365. [CrossRef] [PubMed]
49. Hwang, S.; Kim, E.; Lee, I.; Marcotte, E.M. Systematic comparison of variant calling pipelines using gold standard personal exome variants. *Sci. Rep.* **2015**, *5*, 17875. [CrossRef] [PubMed]
50. Lefterova, M.I.; Shen, P.; Odegaard, J.I.; Fung, E.; Chiang, T.; Peng, G.; Davis, R.W.; Wang, W.; Kharrazi, M.; Schrijver, I.; et al. Next-Generation Molecular Testing of Newborn Dried Blood Spots for Cystic Fibrosis. *J. Mol. Diagn.* **2016**, *18*, 267–282. [CrossRef] [PubMed]
51. Bergougnoux, A.; Délétang, K.; Pommier, A.; Varilh, J.; Houriez, F.; Altieri, J.P.; Koenig, M.; Férec, C.; Claustres, M.; Lalau, G.; et al. Functional characterization and phenotypic spectrum of three recurrent disease-causing deep intronic variants of the *CFTR* gene. *J. Cyst. Fibros.* **2019**, *18*, 468–475. [CrossRef] [PubMed]
52. Boemer, F.; Fasquelle, C.; d'Otreppe, S.; Josse, C.; Dideberg, V.; Segers, K.; Guissard, V.; Capraro, V.; Debray, F.G.; Bours, V. A next-generation newborn screening pilot study: NGS on dried blood spots detects causal mutations in patients with inherited metabolic diseases. *Sci. Rep.* **2017**, *7*, 17641. [CrossRef] [PubMed]
53. Bergougnoux, A.; Boureau-Wirth, A.; Rouzier, C.; Altieri, J.-P.; Verneau, F.; Larrieu, L.; Koenig, M.; Claustres, M.; Raynal, C. A false positive newborn screening result due to a complex allele carrying two frequent CF-causing variants. *J. Cyst. Fibros.* **2016**, *15*, 309–312. [CrossRef]
54. Terlizzi, V.; Castaldo, G.; Salvatore, D.; Lucarelli, M.; Raia, V.; Angioni, A.; Carnovale, V.; Cirilli, N.; Casciaro, R.; Colombo, C.; et al. Genotype-phenotype correlation and functional studies in patients with cystic fibrosis bearing *CFTR* complex alleles. *J. Med. Genet.* **2017**, *54*, 224–235. [CrossRef]
55. Salinas, D.B.; Sosnay, P.R.; Azen, C.; Young, S.; Raraigh, K.S.; Keens, T.G.; Kharrazi, M. Benign and Deleterious Cystic Fibrosis Transmembrane Conductance Regulator Mutations Identified by Sequencing in Positive Cystic Fibrosis Newborn Screen Children from California. *PLoS ONE* **2016**, *11*, e0155624. [CrossRef]

56. Ren, C.L.; Borowitz, D.S.; Gonska, T.; Howenstine, M.S.; Levy, H.; Massie, J.; Milla, C.; Munck, A.; Southern, K.W. Cystic Fibrosis Transmembrane Conductance Regulator-Related Metabolic Syndrome and Cystic Fibrosis Screen Positive, Inconclusive Diagnosis. *J. Pediatr.* **2017**, *181*, S45–S51. [CrossRef]
57. Ooi, C.Y.; Castellani, C.; Keenan, K.; Avolio, J.; Volpi, S.; Boland, M.; Kovesi, T.; Bjornson, C.; Chilvers, M.A.; Morgan, L.; et al. Inconclusive Diagnosis of Cystic Fibrosis After Newborn Screening. *Pediatrics* **2015**, *135*, e1377–e1385. [CrossRef] [PubMed]
58. Munck, A.; Bourmaud, A.; Bellon, G.; Picq, P.; Farrell, P.M.; DPAM Study Group. Phenotype of children with inconclusive cystic fibrosis diagnosis after newborn screening. *Pediatr. Pulmonol.* **2020**, *55*, 918–928. [CrossRef] [PubMed]
59. Thauvin-Robinet, C.; Munck, A.; Huet, F.; Génin, E.; Bellis, G.; Gautier, E.; Audrézet, M.-P.; Férec, C.; Lalau, G.; Georges, M.D.; et al. The very low penetrance of cystic fibrosis for the R117H mutation: A reappraisal for genetic counselling and newborn screening. *J. Med. Genet.* **2009**, *46*, 752–758. [CrossRef] [PubMed]
60. Boussaroque, A.; Audrézet, M.-P.; Raynal, C.; Sermet-Gaudelus, I.; Bienvenu, T.; Férec, C.; Bergougnoux, A.; Lopez, M.; Scotet, V.; Munck, A.; et al. Penetrance is a critical parameter for assessing the disease liability of *CFTR* variants. *J. Cyst. Fibros.* **2020**, in press. [CrossRef]
61. Hayeems, R.Z.; Miller, F.A.; Barg, C.J.; Bombard, Y.; Carroll, J.C.; Tam, K.; Kerr, E.; Chakraborty, P.; Potter, B.K.; Patton, S.; et al. Psychosocial Response to Uncertain Newborn Screening Results for Cystic Fibrosis. *J. Pediatr.* **2017**, *184*, 165–171. [CrossRef]
62. McClaren, B.J.; Metcalfe, S.A.; Aitken, M.; Massie, R.J.; Ukoumunne, O.C.; Amor, D.J. Uptake of carrier testing in families after cystic fibrosis diagnosis through newborn screening. *Eur. J. Hum. Genet.* **2010**, *18*, 1084–1089. [CrossRef]
63. Dequeker, E.; Stuhrmann, M.; Morris, M.A.; Casals, T.; Castellani, C.; Claustres, M.; Cuppens, H.; des Georges, M.; Ferec, C.; Macek, M.; et al. Best practice guidelines for molecular genetic diagnosis of cystic fibrosis and CFTR-related disorders—updated European recommendations. *Eur. J. Hum. Genet.* **2009**, *17*, 51–65. [CrossRef]
64. Castellani, C.; Cuppens, H.; Macek, M.; Cassiman, J.J.; Kerem, E.; Durie, P.; Tullis, E.; Assael, B.M.; Bombieri, C.; Brown, A.; et al. Consensus on the use and interpretation of cystic fibrosis mutation analysis in clinical practice. *J. Cyst. Fibros.* **2008**, *7*, 179–196. [CrossRef]
65. Boussaroque, A.; Bergougnoux, A.; Raynal, C.; Audrézet, M.-P.; Sasorith, S.; Férec, C.; Bienvenu, T.; Girodon, E. Pitfalls in the interpretation of *CFTR* variants in the context of incidental findings. *Hum. Mutat.* **2019**, *40*, 2239–2246. [CrossRef]
66. Ceyhan-Birsoy, O.; Murry, J.B.; Machini, K.; Lebo, M.S.; Yu, T.W.; Fayer, S.; Genetti, C.A.; Schwartz, T.S.; Agrawal, P.B.; Parad, R.B.; et al. Interpretation of Genomic Sequencing Results in Healthy and Ill Newborns: Results from the BabySeq Project. *Am. J. Hum. Genet.* **2019**, *104*, 76–93. [CrossRef]
67. Kingsmore, S.F. Newborn testing and screening by whole-genome sequencing. *Genet. Med.* **2016**, *18*, 214–216. [CrossRef] [PubMed]
68. Wilcken, B.; Wiley, V. Fifty years of newborn screening. *J. Paediatr. Child Health* **2015**, *51*, 103–107. [CrossRef] [PubMed]
69. Nijmeijer, S.C.M.; Conijn, T.; Lakeman, P.; Henneman, L.; Wijburg, F.A.; Haverman, L. Attitudes of the general population towards preconception expanded carrier screening for autosomal recessive disorders including inborn errors of metabolism. *Mol. Genet. Metab.* **2019**, *126*, 14–22. [CrossRef] [PubMed]
70. Delatycki, M.B.; Alkuraya, F.; Archibald, A.; Castellani, C.; Cornel, M.; Grody, W.W.; Henneman, L.; Ioannides, A.S.; Kirk, E.; Laing, N.; et al. International perspectives on the implementation of reproductive carrier screening. *Prenat. Diagn.* **2020**, *40*, 301–310. [CrossRef] [PubMed]
71. Castellani, C.; Picci, L.; Tridello, G.; Casati, E.; Tamanini, A.; Bartoloni, L.; Scarpa, M.; Assael, B.M. Cystic fibrosis carrier screening effects on birth prevalence and newborn screening. *Genet. Med.* **2016**, *18*, 145–151. [CrossRef] [PubMed]
72. Bell, S.C.; Mall, M.A.; Gutierrez, H.; Macek, M.; Madge, S.; Davies, J.C.; Burgel, P.-R.; Tullis, E.; Castaños, C.; Castellani, C.; et al. The future of cystic fibrosis care: A global perspective. *Lancet Respir. Med.* **2020**, *8*, 65–124. [CrossRef]

73. Gruber, A.; Pacault, M.; El Khattabi, L.A.; Vaucouleur, N.; Orhant, L.; Bienvenu, T.; Girodon, E.; Vidaud, D.; Leturcq, F.; Costa, C.; et al. Non-invasive prenatal diagnosis of paternally inherited disorders from maternal plasma: Detection of NF1 and *CFTR* mutations using droplet digital PCR. *Clin. Chem. Lab. Med.* **2018**, *56*, 728–738. [CrossRef]
74. Guissart, C.; Tran Mau Them, F.; Debant, V.; Viart, V.; Dubucs, C.; Pritchard, V.; Rouzier, C.; Boureau-Wirth, A.; Haquet, E.; Puechberty, J.; et al. A Broad Test Based on Fluorescent-Multiplex PCR for Noninvasive Prenatal Diagnosis of Cystic Fibrosis. *Fetal. Diagn. Ther.* **2019**, *45*, 403–412. [CrossRef]

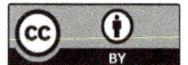
© 2020 by the authors. Licensee MDPI, Basel, Switzerland. This article is an open access article distributed under the terms and conditions of the Creative Commons Attribution (CC BY) license (http://creativecommons.org/licenses/by/4.0/).

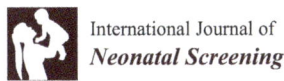

Review

Inconclusive Diagnosis after Newborn Screening for Cystic Fibrosis

Anne Munck

Hopital Necker Enfants-Malades, AP-HP, CF centre, Université Paris Descartes, 75015 Paris, France; anne.munck1@gmail.com; Tel.: +33-60-9372-870

Received: 13 February 2020; Accepted: 10 March 2020; Published: 12 March 2020

Abstract: An unintended consequence of newborn screening for cystic fibrosis (CF) is the identification of infants with a positive screening test but an inconclusive diagnostic testing. These infants are designated as CF transmembrane conductance regulator-related metabolic syndrome (CRMS) in the US and CF screen-positive, inconclusive diagnosis (CFSPID) in Europe. Recently, experts agreed on a unified international definition of CRMS/CFSPID which will improve our knowledge on the epidemiology and outcomes of these infants and optimize comparisons between cohorts. Many of these children will remain free of symptoms, but a number may develop clinical features suggestive of CFTR-related disorder (CFTR-RD) or CF later in life. Clinicians should to be prepared to identify these infants and communicate with parents about this challenging and stressful situation for both healthcare professionals and families. In this review, we present the recent publications on infants designated as CRMS/CFSPID, including the definition, the incidence across Europe, the assessment of the CFTR protein function, the outcomes with the rates of conversion to a final diagnosis of CF and their management.

Keywords: cystic fibrosis; CF transmembrane conductance regulator-related metabolic syndrome; CF screen positive; inconclusive diagnosis; newborn screening

---

1. Introduction

Newborn screening (NBS) for cystic fibrosis (CF), when combined with very early multidisciplinary care at CF centers (CFC), is acknowledged as the optimal approach to CF diagnosis, as it maximizes the long-term prognosis and survival of these children [1–3]. However, beyond the goal of NBS and irrespective of the screening protocol used, there is the detection of infants with a positive NBS test and an inconclusive designation [4]. The terminology used for these infants is CF transmembrane conductance regulator-related metabolic syndrome (CRMS) in the US [5] and CF screen-positive, inconclusive diagnosis (CFSPID) in Europe [6]. Many of these children will remain asymptomatic, but later in life, a number of them may develop symptoms suggestive or CFTR-related disorder (CFTR-RD) or CF [7]. The approach to these infants is evolving as clinical experience grows; nevertheless, uncertainty remains challenging for families and caregivers

2. Inconclusive Diagnosis after Newborn Screening

2.1. Definition of CRMS/CFSPID

For infants with a positive NBS test but an inconclusive diagnosis, a definition has been created using the terminology CRMS in the US since 2009 [5] that is included in the International Statistical Classification of Diseases and Related Health Problems, Ninth Revision medical code (277.9), which is mandatory in the US for healthcare delivery. Recently, in Europe, a Delphi process conducted by the European CF Society (ECFS) Neonatal Screening Working Group (NN WG) identified the need for a designation, and the terminology CFSPID was introduced in 2015 [6]. The differences between these two definitions were minor. To optimize comparisons between cohorts and thus improve our knowledge on the epidemiology and outcomes, experts from around the world gathered at a Diagnosis Consensus Conference held in the US, in 2015, and agreed on a unified definition (Table 1) of CRMS/CFSPID [8], with a recently published algorithm for this definition in Figure 1 [9]. This definition incorporates the knowledge on *CFTR* variants characteristics as "CF causing", "non-CF causing", "varying clinical consequences" or "unknown significance" [10] in the CFTR2 database, which is regularly updated and searchable on the website https://cftr2.org. However, an international survey conducted in 2018 by ECFS NN WG, with support of the Cystic Fibrosis Foundation (CFF) NBS Quality Improvement Group, showed significant confusion in regard to the correct designation of inconclusive diagnosis in six scenarios of infants screening positive. In one-third to half of the respondents, who were either CF doctors or pediatric pulmonologists [9], the diagnosis option was incorrect, thus identifying the need for improved education and communication.

Table 1. Definitions for CF transmembrane conductance regulator-related metabolic syndrome (CRMS) and CF screen-positive, inconclusive diagnosis (CFSPID) and the harmonized definition CRMS/CFSPID.

	Positive NBS	**And**	**Or**
CRMS [5] US	Asymptomatic infants with hypertrypsinemia at birth	Persistently intermediate sweat chloride levels [1] and fewer than 2 CF-causing CFTR mutations	Sweat chloride concentration <30 mmol/L and 2 CFTR mutations with 0 or 1 known to be CF-causing
CFSPID [6] Europe	Asymptomatic infants with hypertrypsinemia at birth	0 or 1 CFTR mutation, plus intermediate sweat chloride (30–59 mmol/L)	2 CFTR mutations, at least 1 of which has unclear phenotypic consequences, plus a normal sweat chloride (<30 mmol/L)
CRMS/CFSPID [8]	Infants with positive newborn screening test	Sweat chloride <30 mmol/L and 2 CFTR mutations with 0 or 1 CF-causing CFTR mutation	Sweat chloride 30–59 mmol/L and 0 or 1 CF-causing CFTR mutation

[1] Sweat chloride levels: 30–59 mmol/L if age < 6 months or 40–59 mmol/L if age ≥6 months.

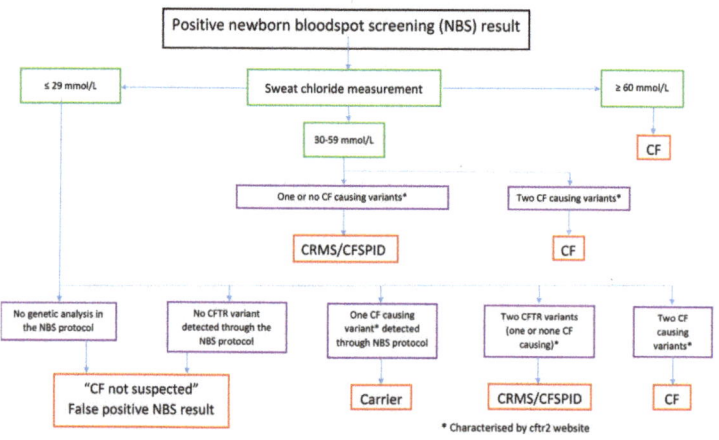

Figure 1. An algorithm for the designation of infants, following the positive newborn screening (NBS) result [9]. CF: Cystic fibrosis, CFTR: CF transmembrane conductance regulator (gene), CFMS: CFTR-related metabolic syndrome, CFSPID: CF screen-positive, inconclusive diagnosis.

2.2. Incidence of CRMS/CFSPID across Europe

Within the two past decades, there has been a huge increase in NBS programs for CF worldwide, including in Europe. A recent European survey [4] reported data from 16 out of the 17 national

NBS protocols with centralized data collection. Since then, national programs have been developed in Portugal (2015), Germany (2016), Denmark (2016), Macedonia (2018) and Belgium (2020); and Spain and Italy have regional programs that provide extensive coverage of the population. Strategies of NBS protocols and structure of programs vary widely, like the proportion of cases designated CRMS/CFSPID, reflecting the different approaches. This survey collected data during the year 2014, when the definition of CFSPID was not yet available, and therefore the recognition of infants may possibly be underestimated. The ratio of infants with CF compared to CFSPID ranged from 1.2:1 (Poland) to 32:1 (Ireland), and protocols, including larger panels of DNA mutations, were more likely to identify those infants. Minimizing the number of cases with CRMS/CFSPID remains an important consideration in NBS programs, as referring and following these infants create a burden for their families and healthcare professionals, and the benefits remain unclear.

2.3. Assessment of CFTR Protein Function

In cases where repeated sweat tests' levels remain within the intermediate range, functional analyses measuring CFTR activity may help clarify the diagnosis. The assessment of the level of CFTR function is based on in vivo pharmacological studies, such as nasal potential difference (NPD) [11] or ex vivo intestinal current measurement (ICM) performed on rectal biopsies perfused in Ussing chambers [12], and on some occasion in combination with intestinal organoids analysis [13]. These evaluations of the CFTR function are performed exclusively in highly specialized CF centers and are not currently used in clinical practice. A diagnosis of CF can be ruled out when these functional analyses are within the normal range. The level of CFTR function further defines the likelihood of developing CF, as there is a continuum of CFTR dysfunction, and the paradigm of CF can be defined in terms of risk, depending on the severity of the dysfunction.

3. Monitoring Infants Designated CRMS/CFSPID

3.1. Outcomes and Conversion to a Final Diagnosis of CF in Infants Designated CRMS/CFSPID

Infants designated CRMS/CFSPID may later develop a diagnosis of CFTR-RD, and a number may have symptoms suggestive of CF and convert to a final diagnosis of CF (a less classical form in most cases). The range of conversion to CF varied widely in retrospective or registry database studies [14–18], from 6% [14] to 48% [15] (Table 2). Neither the definition of cases with an inconclusive diagnosis nor the diagnosis criteria for conversion to CF was consistent among these studies, as well as the duration of follow-up, thus providing an explanation in this wide range of conversion to CF. Reclassification to CF should be based either on subsequent positive sweat test and/or two *CFTR* variants as CF causing *in trans* according to new knowledge acquired in CFTR2. Conversion to CF is also more likely related to individual CFTR variants [19–21] and to infants with an initial intermediate sweat chloride (SC) value compared to normal SC [16]. In two recent prospective studies, the conversion rate varied from 11% [19] to 44% [21]. The first prospective study was set up by Ooi et al. [19] in eight CF centers in Canada and Italy. Eighty-two positive NBS infants with an inconclusive diagnosis of CF, born 2007–2013, were matched 1:1 with a cohort diagnosed with CF through NBS ($n = 80$) and were evaluated at a median age of 2.2 years. Those with a CRMS/CFSPID designation at baseline had significantly lower median IRT (77 µg/L vs. 144 µg/L, $p < 0.0001$) and SC values (27.3 mmol/L vs. 83.2 mmol/L, $p < 0.0001$) compared to those diagnosed with CF. During follow-up, compared to those with CF, they all had sustained exocrine pancreatic sufficiency and less respiratory symptoms as well as identification of *Pseudomonas aeruginosa* (12% vs. 31%) and *Staphylococcus aureus* (40% vs. 70%). Among the 82 cases with a CRMS/CFSPID diagnosis, nine (11%) children converted to a delayed CF diagnosis based on positive SC value ($n = 2$), with the identification of two CF-causing mutations *in trans* in the CFTR2 database at the time of data analysis ($n = 4$) or both in three cases. Serial repeated sweat testing showed a mean age of 21.3 months at the time of conversion in those diagnosed with CF with a positive SC value. Those who converted to CF had higher initial SC values, no clinical or anthropometric differences and a trend toward more *Pseudomonas aeruginosa* identification compared to those who did not convert to CF. Authors shed light on the limited duration of follow-up with a caution in interpretation, as manifestations suggestive of CF may not develop until adolescence or adulthood. The same team [22] analyzed a larger cohort with CRMS/CFSPID and found a difference in initial NBS IRT median values in those with delayed CF ($n = 14$) compared to those who remained CRMS/CFSPID ($n = 83$), respectively with a median [Q1-Q3] of 108.9 (72.3–126.8) vs. 73.7 (60.0–96.0); $p = 0.02$, suggesting IRT initial value and trajectory over time as a potential tool to stratify young infants into high-risk or low-risk groups of developing CF. Munck et al. [21] reported a prospective multicenter study in France. Sixty-three positive NBS infants with an inconclusive diagnosis of CF, born 2002–2009, were matched 1:1 with a cohort diagnosed CF through NBS ($n = 63$) and evaluated at a mean age of 7.4 years. Those with a CRMS/CFSPID designation at baseline had a significantly lower median IRT (97 µg/L vs. 166 µg/L, $p < 0.0001$) and SC values (40 mmol/L vs. 110 mmol/L, $p < 0.0001$) compared to those diagnosed CF. During follow-up, compared to those with CF, they all had sustained exocrine pancreatic sufficiency, less respiratory symptoms and identification of *Pseudomonas aeruginosa* (24% vs. 82%) and *Staphylococcus aureus* (68% vs. 90%). Among the 63 cases with a CRMS/CFSPID diagnosis, 28 (44%) children converted to a delayed CF diagnosis based on a positive SC value ($n = 8$), with the identification of two CF-causing mutations *in trans* in the CFTR2 database at the time of data analysis ($n = 12$) or both in eight cases. All but six presented during follow-up respiratory symptoms suggestive of CF (productive cough, pathogens, antibiotic courses), although not specific to CF. Those who converted to CF had similar initial SC values, no clinical, anthropometric, respiratory pathogens, radiological or spirometry differences at final assessment compared to those who did not convert to CF. Infants recruited in these two studies reflected children currently diagnosed as CRMS/CFSPID, and the conversion to CF was defined by the above strict criteria. Explanations for the discrepancy in CF conversion rates among studies may be a time lag in infants' birth dates with differences in updated CFTR2 knowledge at the time of data analysis, as well as variations in the duration of follow-up.

3.2. Management of Infants with CRMS/CFSPID Designation

Whether screening newborns for CRMS/CFSPID is of clinical benefit has yet to be established, as most of these infants seem unlikely to develop any phenotype. Those designated CRMS/CFSPID have no clinical feature suggestive of CF at initial evaluation. It is important to provide accurate information to parents who feel psychologically distressed with the delivery of an initial positive NBS result and an inconclusive designation [23]. For an appropriate follow-up, most CF physicians agree that a balance is needed to avoid both overmedicalization and undertreatment, which can be a missed opportunity to prevent manifestations later in life. Nevertheless, there is no evidence that early proactive treatment leads to better long-term outcomes. Considering the US guidelines [5] published in 2009 and European recommendations [21,24] published in 2009 and updated in 2015 on early management, they are in agreement on care issues and on regular follow-up by a physician with an interest in CF encouraging clinical assessment rather than unnecessary explorations and including regular sweat testing. Clear information should be provided to the family and the primary care physician over time. Ooi et al. [19] considered his study as an interim one according to the short duration of monitoring and that CF-like manifestations may not develop until adolescence or adulthood. Data of Munck et al. [21], with a longer monitoring period and a more comprehensive respiratory status assessment, support a less intensive approach in the management of these infants compared to those with CF. They consider a possible discharge from the CF center after six years of age if the child has not converted to CF with the primary care physician remaining vigilant, especially for unexplained chronic lung disease. The best practice for monitoring these children is still an unanswered issue. Both prospective studies shed light on the need of further long-term prospective studies. In parallel, the ECFS NN WG is now working on a consensual document for monitoring these individuals from initial assessment to six years of age, with a diagnostic testing section, a care management section, including respiratory phenotype, and a review of evidence from a year-six assessment, with shared a decision on future care plans with the family.

Table 2. Summary of recent studies of CRMS/CFSPID.

	Kharrazi et al. [14]	Groves et al. [15]	Ren et al. [16]	Levy et al. [17]	Terlizzi et al. [18]	Ooi et al. [19]	Munck et al. [21]
Study design	Retrospective	Retrospective case control	CFF registry	Cross sectional	Retrospective	Prospective case control	Prospective case control
Country	USA California	Australia	US	US Wisconsin	Italy Tuscany	Canada, Italy	France
Birth period	2007–2012	1996–2010	2010–2012	1994–2012	2011–2016	2007–2013	2002–2009
Follow up duration (y)	Mean 4.5	10	1	8	Median 0.6	Median 2.2	Mean 7.4
Number CF	345	225	1540	300	32	80	63
Number CRMS/CFSPID	533	29 [2]	309	57	50	82	63 [2]
CF:CRMS/CFSPID	0.65:1	7.8:1	5:1	5.2:1	0.64:1	1.8:1 [6]	6.3:1 [6]
Conversion to CF, N (%)	20 (5.8)	14/29 (48) matched to CF	NA [4]	NA [4]	5 (10)	9 (11)	28(44)
Increased SCC ≥60 mmol/L	17	2 [3]			5	2	8
2 CF causing mutations	0	0			0	4	12
Both criteria	0	0			0	3	8
Other criteria	3	12			0	0	0
Age at conversion (y)	Mean 2.5 ± 1.4				Median 2 (0.2–4)	Mean 1.8 ± 1.2	Unk [1]
Pseudomonas aeruginosa, N (%)	Unk [1]	78.6	10.7	39	25 [5]	12	24
Pancreatic insufficiency, N (%)	3/15 (15)	4/29 (14)	14/309 (4.5)	0	0	0	0
F508del/R117H, N (%)	Unk [1]	4/14 (29)	80/309 (26)	37/57 (63)	0	16/82 (19.5)	27/63 (43)

[1] Unk: unknown; [2] definition slightly different from CRMS/CFSPID; [3] only 8/14 had a repeated sweat test; [4] NA: non-applicable; [5] only 8/50 had swab culture. CF: [6] CF: CRMS/CFSPID ratio from the algorithm. Cystic fibrosis, CFTR: CF transmembrane conductance regulator (gene), CFMS: CFTR-related metabolic syndrome, CFSPID: CF screen-positive, inconclusive diagnosis, SCC: sweat chloride concentration

4. CRMS/CFSPID Registry Database

Analysis of the 2010–2012 CFF Patient Registry database by Ren et al. [15] showed a high rate of misclassification of NBS-positive infants. On one hand, 11% of infants with CRMS had to be reclassified as CF after expansion of the number of CF-causing mutations and/or subsequent positive SC; and on the other hand, 41% of infants with CRMS were assigned as CF, despite not fulfilling the criteria. Now with the unified definition for infants designated CRMS/CFSPID, we can speculate that registry databases monitoring long-term outcomes will provide an accurate assessment of the risk of moving through adolescence or adulthood to CFTR-RD and CF diagnosis and will contribute to better define the modalities of monitoring. The ECFS NN WG is now working with the ECFS Registry team to prepare a European survey for infants with a designation of CRMS/CFSPID, aimed at recording the current situation of existing national or regional registries or databases, or plans and timelines to develop them.

Funding: This research received no external funding.

Acknowledgments: The author would like to thank K.W. Southern, Liverpool, UK, for his agreement to publish in the review Figure 1 and D. Delmas for her technical support.

Conflicts of Interest: The author declares no conflict of interest.

References

1. Dijk, F.N.; Fitzgerald, D.A. The impact of newborn screening and earlier intervention on the clinical course of cystic fibrosis. *Paediatr. Respir. Rev.* **2012**, *13*, 220–225. [CrossRef] [PubMed]
2. Yen, E.H.; Quinton, H.; Borowitz, D. Better nutritional status in early childhood is associated with improved clinical outcomes and survival in patients with cystic fibrosis. *J. Pediatr.* **2013**, *162*, 530–535. [CrossRef] [PubMed]
3. Tridello, G.; Castellani, C.; Meneghelli, I.; Tamanini, A.; Assael, B.M. Early diagnosis from newborn screening maximises survival in severe cystic fibrosis. *ERJ Open Res.* **2018**, *4*, 00109–2017. [CrossRef] [PubMed]
4. Barben, J.; Castellani, C.; Dankert-Roelse, J.; Gartner, S.; Kashirskaya, N.; Linnane, B.; Mayell, S.; Munck, A.; Sands, D.; Sommerburg, O.; et al. The expansion and performance of national newborn screening programmes for cystic fibrosis in Europe. *J. Cyst. Fibros.* **2017**, *16*, 207–213. [CrossRef]
5. Borowitz, D.; Parad, R.B.; Sharp, J.K.; Sabadosa, K.A.; Robinson, K.A.; Rock, M.J.; Farrell, P.M.; Sontag, M.K.; Rosenfeld, M.; Davis, S.D.; et al. Cystic Fibrosis Foundation practice guidelines for the management of infants with cystic fibrosis transmembrane conductance regulator-related metabolic syndrome during the first two years of life and beyond. *J. Pediatr.* **2009**, *155* (Suppl. S6), S106–S116. [CrossRef]
6. Munck, A.; Mayell, S.J.; Winters, V.; Shawcross, A.; Derichs, N.; Parad, R.; Barben, J.; Southern, K.W. ECFS Neonatal Screening Working Group. Cystic Fibrosis Screen Positive, Inconclusive Diagnosis (CFSPID): A new designation and management recommendations for infants with an inconclusive diagnosis following newborn screening. *J. Cyst. Fibros.* **2015**, *14*, 706–713. [CrossRef]
7. Ren, C.L.; Borowitz, D.S.; Gonska, T.; Howenstine, M.S.; Levy, H.; Massie, J.; Milla, C.; Munck, A.; Southern, K.W. Cystic Fibrosis Transmembrane Conductance Regulator-Related Metabolic Syndrome and Cystic Fibrosis Screen Positive, Inconclusive Diagnosis. *J. Pediatr.* **2017**, *181*, S45–S51. [CrossRef]
8. Farrell, P.M.; White, T.B.; Ren, C.L.; Hempstead, S.E.; Accurso, F.; Derichs, N.; Howenstine, M.; McColley, S.A.; Rock, M.; Rosenfeld, M.; et al. Diagnosis of Cystic Fibrosis: Consensus Guidelines from the Cystic Fibrosis Foundation. *J. Pediatr.* **2017**, *181*, S4–S15. [CrossRef]
9. Southern, K.W.; Barben, J.; Gartner, S.; Munck, A.; Castellani, C.; Mayell, S.J.; Davies, J.C.; Winters, V.; Murphy, J.; Salinas, D.; et al. Inconclusive diagnosis after a positive newborn bloodspot screening result for cystic fibrosis; clarification of the harmonised international definition. *J. Cyst. Fibros.* **2019**, *18*, 778–780. [CrossRef]
10. Sosnay, P.R.; Salinas, D.B.; White, T.B.; Ren, C.L.; Farrell, P.M.; Raraigh, K.S.; Girodon, E.; Castellani, C. Applying Cystic Fibrosis Transmembrane Conductance Regulator Genetics and CFTR2 Data to Facilitate Diagnoses. *J. Pediatr.* **2017**, *181*, S27–S32. [CrossRef]

11. Sermet-Gaudelus, I.; Girodon, E.; Roussel, D.; Deneuville, E.; Bui, S.; Huet, F.; Guillot, M.; Aboutaam, R.; Renouil, M.; Munck, A.; et al. Measurement of nasal potential difference in young children with an equivocal sweat test following newborn screening for cystic fibrosis. *Thorax* **2010**, *65*, 539–544. [CrossRef]
12. Derichs, N.; Sanz, J.; Von Kanel, T.; Stolpe, C.; Zapf, A.; Tümmler, B.; Gallati, S.; Ballmann, M. Intestinal current measurement for diagnostic classification of patients with questionable cystic fibrosis: Validation and reference data. *Thorax* **2010**, *65*, 594–599. [CrossRef] [PubMed]
13. De Winter-de Groot, K.M.; Berkers, G.; Marck-van der Wilt, R.E.P.; van der Meer, R.; Vonk, A.; Dekkers, J.F.; Geerdink, M.; Michel, S.; Kruisselbrink, E.; Vries, R.; et al. Forskolin-induced swelling of intestinal organoids correlates with disease severity in adults with cystic fibrosis and homozygous F508del mutations. *J. Cyst. Fibros.* **2019**, in press. [CrossRef] [PubMed]
14. Kharrazi, M.; Yang, J.; Bishop, T.; Lessing, S.; Young, S.; Graham, S.; Pearl, M.; Chow, H.; Ho, T.; Currier, R.; et al. California Cystic Fibrosis Newborn Screening Consortium. Newborn Screening for Cystic Fibrosis in California. *Pediatrics* **2015**, *136*, 1062–1072. [CrossRef] [PubMed]
15. Groves, T.; Robinson, P.; Wiley, V.; Fitzgerald, D.A. Long-term outcomes of children with intermediate sweat chloride values in infancy. *J. Pediatr.* **2015**, *166*, 1469–1474. [CrossRef]
16. Ren, C.L.; Fink, A.K.; Petren, K.; Borowitz, D.S.; McColley, S.A.; Sanders, D.B.; Rosenfeld, M.; Marshall, B.C. Outcomes of infants with indeterminate diagnosis detected by cystic fibrosis newborn screening. *Pediatrics* **2015**, *135*, e1386–e1392. [CrossRef]
17. Levy, H.; Nugent, M.; Schneck, K.; Stachiw-Hietpas, D.; Laxova, A.; Lakser, O.; Rock, M.; Dahmer, M.K.; Biller, J.; Nasr, S.Z.; et al. Refining the continuum of CFTR-associated disorders in the era of newborn screening. *Clin. Genet.* **2016**, *89*, 539–549. [CrossRef]
18. Terlizzi, V.; Mergni, G.; Buzzetti, R.; Centrone, C.; Zavataro, L.; Braggion, C. Cystic fibrosis screen positive inconclusive diagnosis (CFSPID): Experience in Tuscany, Italy. *J. Cyst. Fibros.* **2019**, *18*, 484–490. [CrossRef]
19. Ooi, C.Y.; Castellani, C.; Keenan, K.; Avolio, J.; Volpi, S.; Boland, M.; Kovesi, T.; Bjornson, C.; Chilvers, M.A.; Morgan, L.; et al. Inconclusive diagnosis of cystic fibrosis after newborn screening. *Pediatrics* **2015**, *135*, e1377–e1385. [CrossRef]
20. Salinas, D.B.; Azen, C.; Young, S.; Keens, T.G.; Kharrazi, M.; Parad, R.B. Phenotypes of California CF Newborn Screen-Positive Children with CFTR 5T Allele by TG Repeat Length. *Genet. Test. Mol. Biomark.* **2016**, *20*, 496–503. [CrossRef]
21. Munck, A.; Bourmaud, A.; Bellon, G.; Picq, P.; Farrell, P.M.; DPAM Study Group. Phenotype of children with inconclusive cystic fibrosis diagnosis after newborn screening. *Pediatr. Pulmonol.* **2016**, *20*, 496–503. [CrossRef] [PubMed]
22. Ooi, C.Y.; Sutherland, R.; Castellani, C.; Keenan, K.; Boland, M.; Reisman, J.; Bjornson, C.; Chilvers, M.A.; van Wylick, R.; Kent, S.; et al. Immunoreactive trypsinogen levels in newborn screened infants with an inconclusive diagnosis of cystic fibrosis. *BMC Pediatr.* **2019**, *19*, 369. [CrossRef] [PubMed]
23. Hayeems, R.Z.; Miller, F.A.; Barg, C.J.; Bombard, Y.; Carroll, J.C.; Tam, K.; Kerr, E.; Chakraborty, P.; Potter, B.K.; Patton, S. Psychosocial Response to Uncertain Newborn Screening Results for Cystic Fibrosis. *J. Pediatr.* **2017**, *184*, 165–171. [CrossRef] [PubMed]
24. Mayell, S.J.; Munck, A.; Craig, J.V.; Sermet, I.; Brownlee, K.G.; Schwarz, M.J.; Castellani, C.; Southern, K.W. European Cystic Fibrosis Society Neonatal Screening Working Group. A European consensus for the evaluation and management of infants with an equivocal diagnosis following newborn screening for cystic fibrosis. *J. Cyst. Fibros.* **2009**, *8*, 71–78. [CrossRef]

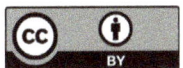

© 2020 by the author. Licensee MDPI, Basel, Switzerland. This article is an open access article distributed under the terms and conditions of the Creative Commons Attribution (CC BY) license (http://creativecommons.org/licenses/by/4.0/).

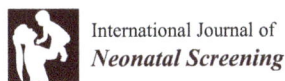

Review

Processing Newborn Bloodspot Screening Results for CF

Jürg Barben [1],* and Jane Chudleigh [2]

[1] Division of Paediatric Pulmonology & CF Centre, Children's Hospital of Eastern Switzerland, 9006 St. Gallen, Switzerland
[2] School of Health Sciences, City, University of London, London EC1V 0HB, UK; j.chudleigh@city.ac.uk
* Correspondence: juerg.barben@kispisg.ch; Tel.: +41-712-437-111; Fax: +41-712-437-699

Received: 6 March 2020; Accepted: 23 March 2020; Published: 25 March 2020

Abstract: Every newborn bloodspot screening (NBS) result for cystic fibrosis (CF) consists of two parts: a screening part in the laboratory and a clinical part in a CF centre. When introducing an NBS programme, more attention is usually paid to the laboratory part, especially which algorithm is most suitable for the region or the country. However, the clinical part, how a positive screening result is processed, is often underestimated and can have great consequences for the affected child and their parents. A clear algorithm for the diagnostic part in CF centres is also important and influences the performance of a CF NBS programme. The processing of a positive screening result includes the initial information given to the parents, the invitation to the sweat test, what to do if a sweat test fails, information about the results of the sweat test, the inconclusive diagnosis and the carrier status, which is handled differently from country to country. The time until the definitive diagnosis and adequate information is given, is considered by the parents and the CF team as the most important factor. The communication of a positive NBS result is crucial. It is not a singular event but rather a process that includes ensuring the appropriate clinicians are aware of the result and that families are informed in the most efficient and effective manner to facilitate consistent and timely follow-up.

Keywords: cystic fibrosis; newborn screening; presumptive diagnosis; sweat test; parental information

1. Introduction

Many countries have now introduced newborn bloodspot screening (NBS) for cystic fibrosis (CF) using a large variety of protocols [1,2]. After proper collection of the dried blood spot specimen, each NBS programme consists of a screening part in the laboratory and a diagnostic part in a CF centre. Most NBS programmes use a 2- or 3-step procedure in the laboratory, with the measurement of immunoreactive trypsinogen (IRT) being the first step [2]. The choice of the second step depends on the presence of CF transmembrane conductance regulator (CFTR) mutations, the health care system and the legislation of a country. Most programs today have CFTR determination as the second step; some use pancreatitis-associated protein (PAP) determination or a second IRT measurement. Therefore, the definition of a positive NBS screening result is handled slightly differently depending on the algorithm used. Like any other screening programme, a positive NBS result requires a confirmatory diagnosis, which for CF is done by means of a sweat test [3]. In accordance with WHO screening guidelines [4], the aim of every NBS programme is to detect children with CF as early as possible and to initiate the appropriate treatment. This means that the sweat test and a clinical evaluation should be performed as soon as possible in an experienced CF centre so that children with a confirmed CF diagnosis can be treated as early as possible. According to the current ECFS guidelines, infants with a confirmed diagnosis after NBS should be seen by the CF specialist team within one month (and no later than 58 days after birth) [3,5]. At the same time, false-positive screening results leading to recalls and sweat tests should be minimised as far as possible. The procedure following a positive NBS result (initial information to parents, invitation to the sweat test, information on the results of the sweat test, inconclusive diagnosis and carrier status) is different from country to country. For parents, the waiting period until the final diagnosis and information adapted to their knowledge is the most important part of the screening process [6]. In a survey of CF specialists, timeliness was also deemed very important by all respondents to ensure that children and their families were seen as soon as possible after receiving the initial positive NBS result [7].

2. Sweat Test—The Gold Standard Confirmation Test of a Positive NBS Result

It has been acknowledged that diagnosing CF is complex and that despite consensus guidelines being published on the diagnosis of CF, there is evidence that these are not applied consistently [3,5]. To confirm a positive NBS result, the determination of chloride concentration in the sweat is still considered the gold standard, because it investigates the function of the chloride channel, which is crucial in CF [8,9]. Most screened infants have little or no clinical manifestation of the disease, making sweat testing the main diagnostic tool to discriminate between children with and without CF [3,5,8,10]. A positive NBS result always requires a confirmatory sweat test, as there may be laboratory errors (mix-up of samples) or the two CFTR mutations detected in the genetic test are on the same allele [3,11]. The diagnostic algorithm of sweat testing is shown in Figure 1 [12].

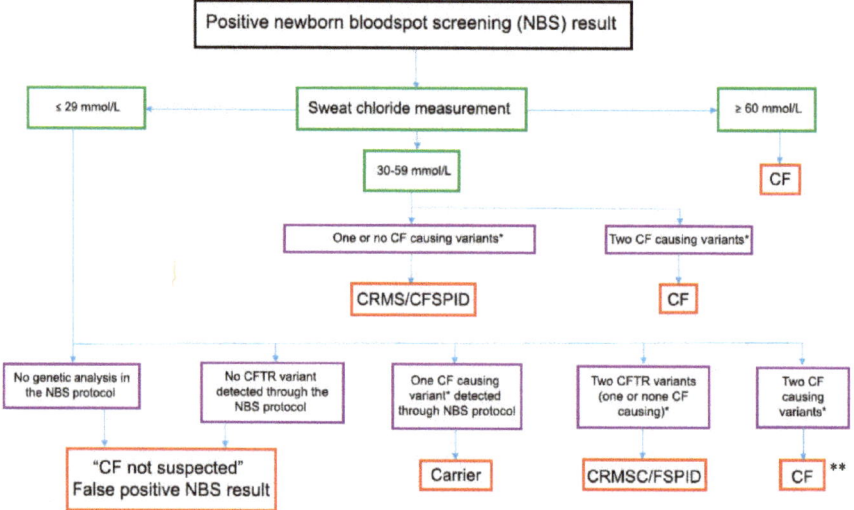

Figure 1. Adapted from reference [12] An algorithm for the designation of infants following a positive newborn bloodspot screening (NBS) result. (CF, cystic fibrosis; CFTR, CF transmembrane conductance regulator (gene); CRMS, CFTR-related metabolic syndrome; CFSPID, CF screen positive, inconclusive diagnosis; CRMS/CFSPID, harmonised definition). * Characterised by the CFTR2 website. ** If two CF causing mutations are present, a repetition of a sweat test is not necessary, but the parents should be genetically tested to exclude the presence of variants in the *cis* form.

However, sweat collection in infants is challenging and must be performed according to current guidelines [9,13,14]. A sufficient amount of sweat is needed to determine the chloride concentration; the smaller the children are or the lighter they are, the more difficult it is to obtain sufficient sweat. A sweat test should not be performed in children <2 kg, and the rates of sweat collections with insufficient volume (called Quantity Not Sufficient, QNS) are below 10% if the child weighs ≥4 kg [15,16]. Collecting sweat from two sites (left and right arm), as is recommended in the US, can reduce the QNS rate. The minimal standards and the diagnostic standards for laboratories performing sweat testing according to the recently revised ECFS best practice guidelines, are listed in Tables 1 and 2 [5].

Table 1. Minimal standards for laboratories performing sweat tests (according to the ECFS Guidelines, adapted from reference [5])

1	Sweat collection by experienced personnel (at least 150 sweat tests per annum) following national or international guidelines and subject to regular (at least annual) peer review.
2	Use of commercially available equipment approved for diagnostic use according to the national regulatory requirements or EU standards if no local ones are available.
3	Internal quality control (usually three samples) with acceptable limits of agreement for chloride before each sweat analysis.
4	Regular external quality assurance for the analyses according to national guidelines.
5	A high number of QNS (Quantity Not Sufficient) rates is a marker of technical issue. This necessitates renewing training for personnel experiencing sweat tests.

Table 2. Diagnostic standards of a sweat test (according to the ECFS Guidelines, adapted from reference [5])

1	The quantity of sweat should indicate an adequate rate of sweat production (15µL for Macroduct™ tube system).
2	The sweat sample should be processed immediately after sweat collection.
3	A sweat chloride value >59 mmol/L is consistent with a diagnosis of CF.
4	A sweat chloride value <30 mmol/L makes the diagnosis of CF unlikely. However, specific CF causing mutations can be associated with a sweat test below 30 mmol/L. These include c.3718-2477C N T (3849 + 10kbC N T) and mutations associated with varied clinical consequence, such as c.617T N G (L206W), c.1040G N A (R347H) and c.3454G N C (D1152H).
5	Individuals with sweat chloride values in the borderline range (30–59 mmol/L) should undergo a repeat sweat test and further evaluation in a specialist CF centre, including detailed clinical assessment and extensive CFTR gene mutation analysis.

The recommendations of the US Cystic Fibrosis Foundation (CFF) say that the proportion of unsuccessful sweat tests in infants should be less than 10% [9,17]. In reality, the failure rate can be as high as 40% during the first three months of life. The rates of QNS samples is higher the earlier you test these children [15,17–20]. More effective NBS protocols have earlier results but higher QNS rates as babies are lighter at the time of testing.

Nowadays, the sweat collection is more frequently undertaken with a capillary tube system (Macroduct™), which was introduced in 1986 and only needs 15 µL of sweat to perform a chloride analysis [21–24]. Measuring conductivity using the Sweat-Check™ analyser has been suggested to be as effective as chloride determination in discriminating healthy children from those with CF [21,25–27]. Nanoduct™ is a newer sweat conductivity analysis system that was specially developed for newborns as it requires only 3–5 µL of sweat and measures conductivity in situ [28]. A few studies have assessed and confirmed its ability to discriminate between those affected by CF and healthy children [16,29–33]. According to current guidelines, conductivity measurement is an accepted method to rule out CF, but for a definite diagnosis, the determination of sweat chloride is required as it is better validated [9,14,24]. As the Nanoduct™ system does not require further laboratory equipment and personnel, it could have a role in remote areas where resources are limited and for ambulatory sweat testing.

3. Presumptive Diagnosis or How to Proceed if a Sweat Test Fails

In some children, a determination of the sweat chlorides is not possible because of too little sweat production (QNS). So far, most algorithms do not explain what to do when sweat tests fail. Sometimes it is delayed until the child is older or heavier and this can take weeks before a sweat test is possible, and can lead to great uncertainty among parents [6]. In the Swiss NBS programme, if a sweat test was not possible, the sweat test was initially repeated after a few weeks or months until it was successful. However, this led to longer waiting times for definite diagnosis, and anxiety among families.

After one year, the algorithm was changed, and genetic testing was directly performed after a sweat test failure. This led to greater detection of unclear cases, now called CF Screen Positive Inconclusive Diagnosis (CFSPID), but no reduction in waiting time. After that, the algorithm was again changed, and measurement of faecal elastase (FE) was introduced that significantly reduced the number of CFSPID infants being identified and improved the timeliness to start pancreatic enzyme replacement therapy (PERT) [34]. This well-documented change in diagnostic procedure highlights the fact that the algorithm for the diagnostic part of the newborn screening used in the CF centres is also important and affects the performance of a CF–NBS programme with regard to the ratio CF:CFSPID and the time until definite diagnosis. In the case of a high clinical probability of a CF diagnosis, one should not wait until the chloride result of a sweat test is available. A positive NBS for CF and a high sweat conductivity make the diagnosis of CF very likely and further investigations (determination of faecal elastase, confirm CFTR variants if necessary) should be initiated at first clinical visit. If symptoms such as lack of weight gain or steatorrhoea are present, start of PERT and salt supplements should not be delayed. A possible pathway is shown in Figure 2. In case of two CFTR variants and a negative sweat test the parents should be genetically tested to exclude the presence of variants in *cis* form. The definite confirmation of the diagnosis with a sweat chloride measurement should be performed at a later stage, as soon as the child reaches a higher weight (>4000g) [34]. This is also important because in the future, sweat chloride values will be a surrogate marker to determine the effect of CFTR modulators in early childhood.

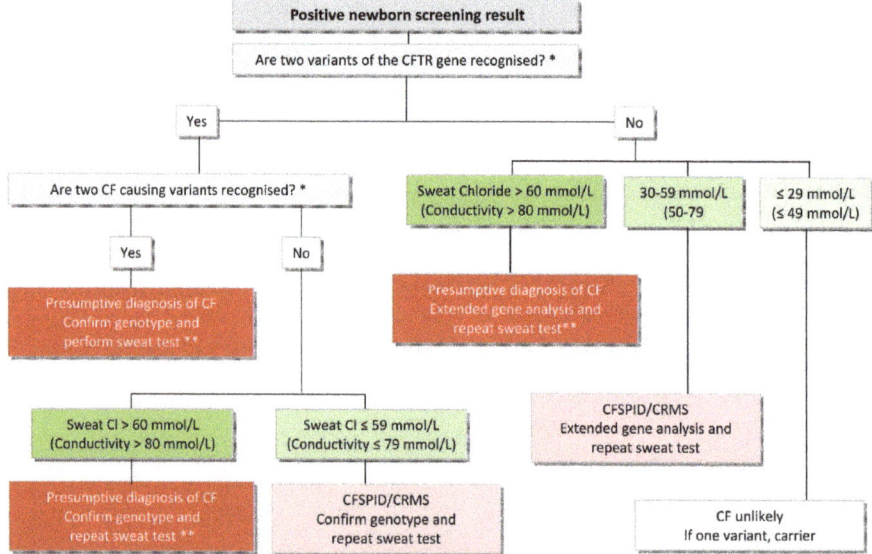

Figure 2. Diagnostic algorithm after a positive NBS result in the CF centre. * According to the CFTR2 website. ** Infants at this point have a presumptive diagnosis of CF and treatment should be established. Further testing is required to consolidate the diagnosis.

4. Unintended Effects of Newborn Screening for CF

Depending on the algorithm chosen, NBS for CF results in recognition of unclear cases, now called CFSPID. Evaluation and management of these infants can be quite challenging [35,36]. This is especially the case if the second step in the screening algorithm is to search for a large number of CFTR mutations whose clinical relevance is different or not yet known. Depending on the chosen algorithm in the diagnostic process in a CF centre, there are also more and more unclear cases [34]. These children have in most cases a favourable prognosis and there is no evidence for improvement through early treatment [37]. In these unclear cases, the disadvantages of early detection with unnecessary medicalisation and burden to the family may outweigh the benefits of early detection [38].

False-positive results are a challenge to every screening programme, since they cause parental anxiety and unnecessary medical examinations [39,40]. NBS programmes using DNA analysis in their algorithm have improved specificity but identify heterozygote carriers, which can cause some anxiety and depression in affected families [6].

False negative results are also a challenge for screening programmes, as parents may feel reassured that the screening did not show a positive result and may consider that CF has been ruled out and possibly be less likely to go to the doctor later if the symptoms are present. Even in the best performing NBS programmes, some CF-affected individuals will be missed. The extent depends on the chosen cut-off value of the initial IRT measurement (false negatives in up to 8%) and the selected algorithm in the screening phase, and needs to be balanced with achieving a reasonable positive predicted value (PPV). Children with meconium ileus may have a negative NBS result, but always require an assessment with sweat and genetic testing.

5. Consequences for Other Family Members

Once a CF diagnosis has been confirmed (or ruled out), the parents and other family members may be offered genetic screening and counselling. All siblings of a positively screened child need to be screened for CF with a sweat test. Asymptomatic adult family members may wish to be screened for carrier status to allow them to make informed choices about reproduction planning and prenatal screening. Adequate genetic counselling should also be arranged or made available to them.

6. Communicating Positive NBS Results for CF

Providing clear information to families is an important part of the NBS process to minimise unnecessary stress and anxiety. To date, there is no internationally accepted approach on how best to do this [7]. Communicating positive NBS results for any condition is not an event but a process that starts with the moment the result is identified as being above the agreed "cut off" and ends when the parents are given the definitive diagnosis for their child [41]. As a positive NBS result in itself is not diagnostic, and further tests are required to confirm or refute the NBS result before a definitive diagnosis is given to the family, this presents a period of uncertainty for families. This may be exacerbated in NBS for CF due to the range of possible outcomes, including a carrier result, confirmation of a diagnosis of CF or a designation of CFSPID, and the wide clinical spectrum that particularly the latter two presents.

Well-informed parents are less stressed by the screening process [6,39,40,42,43]. NBS programmes debate the antenatal information about the screened diseases in an NBS programme that should be given to new parents, who are already overloaded with information and brochures. In Switzerland, some parents felt that details about the screening test and the disease were missing when they were invited by phone for diagnostic evaluation. But information provided during this phone call is deliberately minimal without mentioning the respective disease, so as to reduce parental anxiety before they receive accurate information from a specialist [6].

When children with a positive NBS results are tested in a CF centre, their parents can feel anxious and depressed whilst awaiting definitive results [39,40]. CF specialists should be aware of the effect of the initial information given to parents and later in the CF centres, since this information can either reassure or cause anxiety to parents. The period between informing parents about a positive screening result and their appointment at the CF centre should be as short as possible. Parents should only be contacted when an appointment can be offered the following day.

According to the current ECFS best practice guidelines [5], a CF specialist should discuss a confirmed or inconclusive CF diagnosis in person with the parents (and not on the phone), and the family should receive written information to read after the consultation. Detailed information should also be sent to the family doctor or paediatrician. Families should be informed of further procedures and controls, the function and achievements of the CF research and made aware of opportunities for participation in clinical trials. In the case of a child identified to be a CF carrier, the family should receive a verbal report of the result, and written information should be sent to the family doctor or paediatrician. This information should be clear that (1) the infant does not have CF, (2) the baby is a healthy carrier of this mutation, (3) future pregnancies for the parents are not free of risk of CF and the parents may opt for genetic counselling, and (4) there are implications that could affect reproductive decision making for extended family members and the infant when they are of child-bearing age. A recently published US epidemiological study concluded that CF-related conditions, such as pancreatitis, infertility, diabetes, etc., were more prevalent among carriers than controls, whereas the individual-level risk remained low for most conditions [44]. This could have implications for future genetic counselling, but until these results are confirmed by other studies in other countries, CF carriers should not be medicalised unnecessarily.

A Swiss study exploring parents' perspective of NBS for CF found that parental dissatisfaction with the communication of the NBS result was associated with poor information provision about the NBS result and the actual disease, again demonstrating the importance of ensuring the information is delivered by someone who is well-informed [6]. An international study with CF clinicians found that in the EU, Australia and New Zealand, a range of professionals are responsible for communicating the positive NBS to families, including midwives, the CF centre, the CF nurse, the NBS laboratory as well as the primary care physician, which had the potential to influence the quality of the information provided to the family [7].

Regardless of who is responsible for communicating the positive NBS result for CF, provision of complete and accurate information reduced parental anxiety and facilitated better decision making regarding seeking diagnostic testing and support from the CF team thereafter. Therefore, whoever is responsible for the initial communication with families should have condition-specific knowledge and be familiar with the NBS algorithm being used [7].

7. Feedback and Tracking

Monitoring the performance of NBS is important as it ensures compliance with relevant guidelines and a high standard of care [5]. This requires good data collection to assess the success of the screening. Many countries have already implemented formal mechanisms to ensure that children are seen in time and that specific protocols are followed, and they report their quality and compliance data [2]. However, as the protocols and associated reported variables differ, it is difficult to draw comparisons between programmes.

In some countries, the process of following up a positive NBS result is less straightforward, which poses difficulties and concerns for CF clinicians. Data from an international study with CF clinicians highlighted concerns in certain countries (particularly Turkey and Germany) regarding ensuring all children who received a positive NBS result received the appropriate diagnostic testing and were followed up in a timely manner by the CF team [7]. This was attributed to the mechanisms in place for communicating the positive NBS result for CF to the child's family. In Germany, the NBS laboratory informs the birth clinic who then informs the parents about their child's positive NBS result. In Turkey, processes were governed by who was seen to "own" the information about the positive NBS result, which in turn determined who was responsible for communicating the positive NBS result to the family. This was considered to have the potential to influence parental perceptions of the urgency and/or necessity for their child to be followed up by the CF team. In addition, in Turkey and Germany, parents are expected to arrange the sweat test after they have been informed of their child's positive NBS result. In Germany, this was due to legal requirements that meant the CF centre could not be sent patient details. This raised concerns for CF clinicians in terms of ensuring that all babies who have a positive NBS result have a sweat test and are seen by the CF team in a timely manner.

8. Conclusions

Processing of a positive NBS screening result for CF has an important role in the success of a CF NBS programme, which is often underestimated when working out the optimal screening algorithm in the laboratory. It is a complex process not least because of the range of possible outcomes and the clinical uncertainty that this can present. Guidelines exist to assist clinicians but there is evidence these are used inconsistently for a range of reasons, including geographical, logistical, legal, financial and cultural constraints. Communication of positive NBS results is also challenging for many of the same reasons and presents a process rather than a singular event. However, whatever process is adopted must ensure this happens consistently and in a timely manner. Complete international harmonisation of NBS for CF is neither practical nor desirable but whatever processes are adopted must ensure outcomes for children, families and clinicians that are commensurate between programmes.

Funding: This research received no external funding.

Conflicts of Interest: The authors declare no conflict of interest.

References

1. Castellani, C.; Massie, J.; Sontag, M.; Southern, K.W. Newborn screening for cystic fibrosis. *Lancet Respir. Med.* **2016**, *4*, 653–661. [CrossRef]
2. Barben, J.; Castellani, C.; Dankert-Roelse, J.; Gartner, S.; Kashirskaya, N.; Linnane, B.; Mayell, S.; Munck, A.; Sands, D.; Sommerburg, O.; et al. The expansion and performance of national newborn screening programmes for cystic fibrosis in Europe. *J. Cyst. Fibros.* **2017**, *16*, 207–213. [CrossRef] [PubMed]
3. Castellani, C.; Southern, K.W.; Brownlee, K.; Roelse, J.D.; Duff, A.; Farrell, M.; Mehta, A.; Munck, A.; Pollitt, R.; Sermet-Gaudelus, I.; et al. European best practice guidelines for cystic fibrosis neonatal screening. *J. Cyst. Fibros.* **2010**, *8*, 153–173. [CrossRef] [PubMed]
4. Wilson, J.M.G.; Jungner, G. *Principles and Practice of Screening for Disease*; Public Health papers, No.34; World Health Organization: Geneva, Switzerland, 1968.
5. Castellani, C.; Duff, A.J.; Bell, S.C.; Heijerman, H.G.; Munck, A.; Ratjen, F.; Sermet-Gaudelus, I.; Southern, K.W.; Barben, J.; Flume, P.A.; et al. ECFS best practice guidelines: The 2018 revision. *J. Cyst. Fibros.* **2018**, *17*, 153–178. [CrossRef] [PubMed]
6. Rueegg, C.S.; Barben, J.; Hafen, G.M.; Moeller, A.; Jurca, M.; Fingerhut, R.; Kuehni, C.E.; Group, T.S.C.F.S. Newborn screening for cystic fibrosis—The parent perspective. *J. Cyst. Fibros.* **2016**, *15*, 443–451. [CrossRef] [PubMed]
7. Chudleigh, J.; Ren, C.L.; Barben, J.; Southern, K.W. International approaches for delivery of positive newborn bloodspot screening results for CF. *J. Cyst. Fibros.* **2019**, *18*, 614–621. [CrossRef]
8. Farrell, P.M.; Rosenstein, B.J.; White, T.B.; Accurso, F.J.; Castellani, C.; Cutting, G.R.; Durie, P.R.; LeGrys, V.A.; Massie, J.; Parad, R.B.; et al. Guidelines for diagnosis of cystic fibrosis in newborns through older adults: Cystic Fibrosis Foundation consensus report. *J. Pediatr.* **2008**, *153*, S4–S14. [CrossRef]
9. LeGrys, V.A.; Yankaskas, J.R.; Quittell, L.M.; Marshall, B.C.; Mogayzel, P.J., Jr.; Cystic Fibrosis Foundation. Diagnostic sweat testing: The Cystic Fibrosis Foundation guidelines. *J. Pediatr.* **2007**, *151*, 85–89. [CrossRef]
10. Farrell, P.M.; White, T.B.; Ren, C.L.; Hempstead, S.E.; Accurso, F.; Derichs, N.; Howenstine, M.; McColley, S.A.; Rock, M.; Rosenfeld, M.; et al. Diagnosis of Cystic Fibrosis: Consensus Guidelines from the Cystic Fibrosis Foundation. *J. Pediatr.* **2017**, *181*, S4–S15. [CrossRef]
11. Bergougnoux, A.; Boureau-Wirth, A.; Rouzier, C.; Altieri, J.P.; Verneau, F.; Larrieu, L.; Koenig, M.; Claustres, M.; Raynal, C. A false positive newborn screening result due to a complex allele carrying two frequent CF-causing variants. *J. Cyst. Fibros.* **2016**, *15*, 309–312. [CrossRef]
12. Southern, K.W.; Barben, J.; Gartner, S.; Munck, A.; Castellani, C.; Mayell, S.J.; Davies, J.C.; Winters, V.; Murphy, J.; Salinas, D.; et al. Inconclusive diagnosis after a positive newborn bloodspot screening result for cystic fibrosis; clarification of the harmonised international definition. *J. Cyst. Fibros.* **2019**, *18*, 780. [CrossRef] [PubMed]
13. CLSI. *Sweat Testing: Sample Collection and Quantitative Chloride Analysis Approved Guideline*, 3rd ed.; Clinical and Laboratory Standards Institute: Wayne, PA, USA, 2009.

14. Royal College of Paediatrics and Child Health. Guidelines for the Performance of the Sweat Test for the Investigation of Cystic Fibrosis in the UK (Version 2). An Evidence Based Guideline 2014. Available online: http://www.acb.org.uk/docs/default-source/committees/scientific/guidelines/acb/sweat-guideline-v2-1.pdf (accessed on 25 March 2020).
15. Eng, W.; LeGrys, V.A.; Schechter, M.S.; Laughon, M.M.; Barker, P.M. Sweat-testing in preterm and full-term infants less than 6 weeks of age. *Pediatric Pulmonol.* **2005**, *40*, 64–67. [CrossRef] [PubMed]
16. Rueegg, C.S.; Kuehni, C.E.; Gallati, S.; Jurca, M.; Jung, A.; Casaulta, C.; Barben, J. Swiss Cystic Fibrosis Screening Group Comparison of two sweat test systems for the diagnosis of cystic fibrosis in newborns. *Pediatric Pulmonol.* **2019**, *54*, 264–272. [CrossRef]
17. LeGrys, V.A.; McColley, S.A.; Li, Z.; Farrell, P.M. The need for quality improvement in sweat testing infants after newborn screening for cystic fibrosis. *J. Pediatr.* **2010**, *157*, 1035–1037. [CrossRef]
18. Kleyn, M.; Korzeniewski, S.; Grigorescu, V.; Young, W.; Homnick, D.; Goldstein-Filbrun, A.; Schuen, J.; Nasr, S. Predictors of insufficient sweat production during confirmatory testing for cystic fibrosis. *Pediatric Pulmonol.* **2011**, *46*, 23–30. [CrossRef] [PubMed]
19. Laguna, T.A.; Lin, N.; Wang, Q.; Holme, B.; McNamara, J.; Regelmann, W.E. Comparison of quantitative sweat chloride methods after positive newborn screen for cystic fibrosis. *Pediatric Pulmonol.* **2012**, *47*, 736–742. [CrossRef] [PubMed]
20. Parad, R.B.; Comeau, A.M.; Dorkin, H.L.; Dovey, M.; Gerstle, R.; Martin, T.; O'Sullivan, B.P. Sweat testing infants detected by cystic fibrosis newborn screening. *J. Pediatr.* **2008**, *147*, S69–S72. [CrossRef] [PubMed]
21. Mastella, G.; Di Cesare, G.; Borruso, A.; Menin, L.; Zanolla, L. Reliability of sweat-testing by the Macroduct collection method combined with conductivity analysis in comparison with the classic Gibson and Cooke technique. *Acta Paediatr.* **2000**, *89*, 933–937. [CrossRef]
22. Baumer, J.H. Evidence based guidelines for the performance of the sweat test for the investigation of cystic fibrosis in the UK. *Arch. Dis. Child.* **2003**, *88*, 1126–1127. [CrossRef]
23. Cole, D.E.; Boucher, M.J. Use of a new sample-collection device (Macroduct) in anion analysis of human sweat. *Clin. Chem.* **1986**, *32*, 1375–1378. [CrossRef]
24. Coakley, J.; Scott, S.; Doery, J.; Greaves, R.; Talsma, P.; Whitham, E.; Winship, J. Australasian Guideline (2nd Edition): An Annex to the CLSI and UK Guidelines for the Performance of the Sweat Test for the Diagnosis of Cystic Fibrosis. *Clin. Biochem. Rev.* **2017**, *38*, 115–130.
25. Hammond, K.B.; Nelson, L.; Gibson, L.E. Clinical evaluation of the macroduct sweat collection system and conductivity analyzer in the diagnosis of cystic fibrosis. *J. Pediatr.* **1994**, *124*, 255–260. [CrossRef]
26. Heeley, M.E.; Woolf, D.A.; Heeley, A.F. Indirect measurements of sweat electrolyte concentration in the laboratory diagnosis of cystic fibrosis. *Arch. Dis. Child.* **2000**, *82*, 420–424. [CrossRef] [PubMed]
27. Lezana, J.L.; Vargas, M.H.; Karam-Bechara, J.; Aldana, R.S.; Furuya, M.E.Y. Sweat conductivity and chloride titration for cystic fibrosis diagnosis in 3834 subjects. *J Cyst. Fibros.* **2003**, *2*, 1–7. [CrossRef]
28. Webster, H.L.; Quirante, C.G. Micro-flowcell conductometric sweat analysis for cystic fibrosis diagnosis. *Ann. Clin. Biochem.* **2000**, *37*, 399–407. [CrossRef]
29. Barben, J.; Ammann, R.A.; Metlagel, A.; Schöni, M.H. Conductivity determined by a new sweat analyzer compared with chloride concentrations for the diagnosis of cystic fibrosis. *J. Pediatr.* **2005**, *146*, 183–188. [CrossRef]
30. Desax, M.C.; Ammann, R.A.; Hammer, J.; Schoeni, M.H.; Barben, J. Nanoduct sweat testing for rapid diagnosis in newborns, infants and children with cystic fibrosis. *Eur. J. Pediatr.* **2008**, *167*, 299–304. [CrossRef]
31. Sands, D.; Oltarzewski, M.; Nowakowska, A.; Zybert, K. Bilateral sweat tests with two different methods as a part of cystic fibrosis newborn screening (CF NBS) protocol and additional quality control. *Folia Histochem. Cytobiol.* **2010**, *48*, 358–365. [CrossRef]
32. Sezer, R.G.; Aydemir, G.; Akcan, A.B.; Paketci, C.; Karaoglu, A.; Aydinoz, S.; Bozaykut, A. Nanoduct sweat conductivity measurements in 2664 patients: Relationship to age, arterial blood gas, serum electrolyte profiles and clinical diagnosis. *J. Clin. Med. Res.* **2013**, *5*, 34–41. [CrossRef]
33. Vernooij-van Langen, A.; Dompeling, E.; Yntema, J.B.; Arets, B.; Tiddens, H.; Loeber, G.; Dankert-Roelse, J. Clinical evaluation of the Nanoduct sweat test system in the diagnosis of cystic fibrosis after newborn screening. *Eur. J. Pediatr.* **2015**, *174*, 1025–1034. [CrossRef]

34. Barben, J.; Rueegg, C.S.; Jurca, M.; Spalinger, J.; Kuehni, C.E.; Swiss Cystic Fibrosis Screening Group. Measurement of fecal elastase improves performance of newborn screening for cystic fibrosis. *J. Cyst. Fibros.* **2016**, *15*, 313–317. [CrossRef] [PubMed]
35. Munck, A.; Mayell, S.J.; Winters, V.; Shawcross, A.; Derichs, N.; Parad, R.; Barben, J.; Southern, K.W. Cystic Fibrosis Screen Positive, Inconclusive Diagnosis (CFSPID): A new designation and management recommendations for infants with an inconclusive diagnosis following newborn screening. *J. Cyst. Fibros.* **2015**, *14*, 706–713. [CrossRef] [PubMed]
36. Ooi, C.Y.; Castellani, C.; Keenan, K.; Avolio, J.; Volpi, S.; Boland, M.; Kovesi, T.; Bjornson, C.; Chilvers, M.A.; Morgan, L.; et al. Inconclusive diagnosis of cystic fibrosis after newborn screening. *Pediatrics* **2015**, *135*, e1377–e1385. [CrossRef] [PubMed]
37. Barben, J.; Southern, K.W. Cystic Fibrosis Screen Positive, inconclusive Diagnosis (CFSPID). *Curr. Opin. Pulm. Med.* **2016**, *22*, 617–622. [CrossRef]
38. Massie, J.; Gillam, L. Uncertain diagnosis after newborn screening for cystic fibrosis: An ethics-based approach to a clinical dilemma. *Pediatric Pulmonol.* **2014**, *49*, 1–7. [CrossRef] [PubMed]
39. Tluczek, A.; Mischler, E.H.; Farrell, P.M.; Fost, N.; Peterson, N.M.; Carey, P.; Bruns, W.T.; McCarthy, C. Parents' knowledge of neonatal screening and response to false-positive cystic fibrosis testing. *J. Dev. Behav. Pediatr.* **1992**, *13*, 181–186. [CrossRef]
40. Tluczek, A.; Koscik, R.L.; Farrell, P.M.; Rock, M.J. Psychosocial risk associated with newborn screening for cystic fibrosis: Parents' experience while awaiting the sweat-test appointment. *Pediatrics* **2005**, *115*, 1692–1703. [CrossRef]
41. Chudleigh, J.; Chinnery, H.; Bonham, J.R.; Olander, E.K.; Moody, L.; Simpson, A.; Morris, S.; Ulph, F.; Bryon, M.; Southern, K.W. *A Qualitative Exploration of Health Professionals' Experiences of Communicating Positive Newborn Bloodspot Screening Results for Nine Conditions in England*; 2020. (In Press)
42. Dillard, J.P.; Shen, L.; Robinson, J.D.; Farrell, P.M. Parental information seeking following a positive newborn screening for cystic fibrosis. *J. Health Commun.* **2010**, *15*, 880–894. [CrossRef]
43. Ulph, F.; Cullinan, T.; Qureshi, N.; Kai, J. Informing children of their newborn screening carrier result for sickle cell or cystic fibrosis: Qualitative study of parents' intentions, views and support needs. *J. Genet. Couns.* **2014**, *23*, 409–420. [CrossRef]
44. Miller, A.C.; Comellas, A.P.; Hornick, D.B.; Stoltz, D.A.; Cavanaugh, J.E.; Gerke, A.K.; Welsh, M.J.; Zabner, J.; Polgreen, P.M. Cystic fibrosis carriers are at increased risk for a wide range of cystic fibrosis-related conditions. *Proc. Natl. Acad. Sci. USA* **2020**, *117*, 1621–1627. [CrossRef]

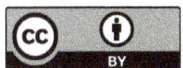

© 2020 by the authors. Licensee MDPI, Basel, Switzerland. This article is an open access article distributed under the terms and conditions of the Creative Commons Attribution (CC BY) license (http://creativecommons.org/licenses/by/4.0/).

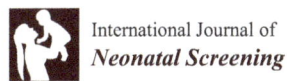

Review
Psychological Impact of NBS for CF

Jane Chudleigh [1,*] and Holly Chinnery [2]

1. School of Health Sciences, City, University of London, London EC1V 0HB, UK
2. Faculty of Sports, Health and Applied Science, St Mary's University, London TW1 4SX, UK; holly.chinnery@stmarys.ac.uk
* Correspondence: j.chudleigh@city.ac.uk

Received: 31 January 2020; Accepted: 25 March 2020; Published: 30 March 2020

Abstract: Newborn screening for cystic fibrosis has resulted in diagnosis often before symptoms are recognised, leading to benefits including reduced disease severity, decreased burden of care, and lower costs. The psychological impact of this often unsought diagnosis on the parents of seemingly well children is less well understood. The time during which the screening result is communicated to families but before the confirmatory test results are available is recognised as a period of uncertainty and it is this uncertainty that can impact most on parents. Evidence suggests this may be mitigated against by ensuring the time between communication and confirmatory testing is minimized and health professionals involved in communicating positive newborn screening results and diagnostic results for cystic fibrosis to families are knowledgeable and able to provide appropriate reassurance. This is particularly important in the case of false positive results or when the child is given a Cystic Fibrosis Screen Positive, Inconclusive Diagnosis designation. However, to date, there are no formal mechanisms in place to support health professionals undertaking this challenging role, which would enable them to meet the expectations set out in specific guidance.

Keywords: newborn bloodspot screening; cystic fibrosis; psychological impact

1. Introduction

The increased use globally of newborn bloodspot screening (NBS) for cystic fibrosis (CF) has resulted in diagnosis often before symptoms are recognised. Benefits include reduced disease severity, decreased burden of care, and lower costs [1–5]. Without NBS, the diagnosis of CF relies on the recognition of particular clinical signs and symptoms, which often results in delayed diagnosis. This can lead to an arduous journey for parents characterised by uncertainty and anxiety as they seek answers and are referred to a number of different clinical specialities before the correct, definitive diagnosis is made [6].

NBS for CF may pose different challenges when compared to other conditions included in NBS programmes, such as sickle cell disease (SCD) which commonly includes antenatal screening, meaning that parents are aware of their own carrier status and the theoretical risk to their unborn child [7]. For CF, parents are often unaware and have not sought information regarding their own carrier status [8]. However, other challenges, such as the method and content of communication, may be similar between conditions.

Despite the undisputed clinical and fiscal benefits of CF NBS, several challenges have been noted, one of which being the potential psychological impact on the child's family. One small study consisting of qualitative interviews with the parents of children diagnosed with CF either via NBS, prenatally, or after the development of symptoms suggested that for those diagnosed via NBS, the early, unsought diagnosis had the potential to deeply affect parents in many ways. These included questioning their competence to care for their baby and their sense of who the baby is. In addition, early diagnosis led to the disease taking centre stage during the child's early weeks and months and caused health professionals to loom very large in the family's life at this formative time [9]. Another study in the US, which explored the parental experiences associated with receiving a positive NBS result for one of the metabolic conditions, supported these findings and suggested that the methods used to communicate the NBS result and the condition specific knowledge of the individual imparting the result influenced parental dissatisfaction, anxiety, and distress [10]. The similarities between the findings of these studies perhaps reflect the fact that CF and the metabolic conditions have a genetic origin and therefore staff knowledge and understanding about the cause and immediate and longer term implications of these are vital.

Like all conditions, it is important that careful consideration is given to how positive CF NBS results are communicated to parents as this is often unexpected, represents a life limiting diagnosis for the child and often a life changing event for the parents. As for many conditions, it may not be possible to remove parental anguish completely from what is an upsetting time. However, it is important for health professionals to communicate positive CF NBS results in a manner that minimises potential distress and does not detrimentally affect parents' relationships with their child and other family members. This chapter will focus on the psychological impact of CF, with implications not always limited to CF, and will explore the current guidance regarding communication strategies, the impact of poor communication practices, and information giving in times of uncertainty, and make recommendations for future practice.

2. Guidance Regarding Communication of Positive NBS Results for CF

Internationally, detailed guidelines exist for the processing of positive CF NBS results [11,12]. However, these primarily focus on laboratory processes and subsequent clinical management; less attention is given to how positive CF NBS results should be communicated to families to minimise potential distress. The European best practice guidelines for CF neonatal screening [3] recognise the time period during which the screening result is communicated to families but before the confirmatory test results are available, as a "period of maximal uncertainty." It is therefore suggested that during this time, information should be provided to families in a format that will be easy for them to digest, using language the family can understand. In addition, information should be structured, clarified, and summarised appropriately and parental understanding should be checked and questions encouraged. These guidelines also suggest the health professional communicating the NBS result should explore the families' beliefs, concerns, and expectations in order to tailor information and the conversation style for the needs of the parent(s). Moreover, in anticipation of further communication needs, the health professional should encourage parental participation in decisions and enlist resources and appropriate support. Finally, health professionals informing parents of their child's positive CF NBS result should be knowledgeable about CF, NBS principles, basic CF genetics, and the psychosocial pitfalls that some parents may experience [3].

More specific guidance from the United Kingdom states that families should be informed by an initial structured telephone call undertaken by a well-informed health professional with appropriate experience and support to give bad news [13]. European guidelines recognise the importance of CF team members possessing compassionate communication and effective information giving skills and the ability to recognise and respond to emotional distress. In addition, these guidelines suggest that some CF team members may require training in more specific skills, such as breaking bad news, recognising significant psychopathology, and appropriate referral should such instances occur. The advantages of the inclusion of specialist mental health professionals in CF teams, such as clinical psychologists or psychiatrists, is also recognised [12].

3. Impact of Communicating Positive NBS Results to Families

In 2015, a systematic review summarised if, and how, information provision has been included in economic evaluations of NBS programmes [14]. This review highlighted that only three studies included an estimate of the cost of information provision in their analysis and none of the studies captured the impact of information provision after screening [14]. One study in the systematic review [14] referred to costs related to the impact of poor information provision specifically related to false positive results rather than poor information provision at the time of communicating the initial NBS+ result per se [15]. This review concluded that evidence existed to support the notion that poor information provision in relation to NBS does impact on parents but there have been few attempts to quantify the impact of information provision in economic evaluations of NBS to date. Importantly, this review confirmed that there are no current data on the long-term impact of poor information provision and subsequent use of healthcare resources and impact on parents' health and well-being. This is interesting since the provision of adequate information and therefore good parental knowledge about their child's false positive CF NBS result, meant that the number of visits to the child's General Practitioner did not differ significantly between the false positive and the negative NBS groups [16]. Therefore, there is clearly a need to explore the role of information provision on the subsequent healthcare resource use.

Studies that have focused on CF NBS have identified adverse outcomes associated with the approaches and methods used to communicate CF NBS results to families. Interviews with the mothers ($n = 106$) and fathers ($n = 97$) of children with a confirmed diagnosis of congenital hypothyroidism (CHT) ($n = 37$), CF-carrier ($n = 43$), or CF ($n = 26$) in the United States (US) found that the majority of parents across all groups reported strong initial emotional reactions such as shock, panic, and anxiety about what results meant. The responses are likely related to the fact that currently, antenatal screening for CHT and CF is not routinely undertaken, therefore parents are unaware of the potential risk of their unborn baby being affected by these conditions. Responses related to positive CF NBS results included fears of the child dying, parental somatic symptoms, such as nausea and suffocation, difficulty bonding with their infant, marital discord, and changed reproductive plans [17]. These differences may reflect the fact that while CHT is treatable with a very good prognosis when diagnosed and treated in infancy, CF continues to be a life-limiting condition with no cure. In addition, in the majority of cases, CHT does not have a genetic origin and therefore does not have the same reproductive implications as CF. A similar study conducted in the US explored factors affecting parent–child relationships one year after positive NBS with 131 mothers and 118 fathers of 131 infants who had a positive NBS result for CF ($n = 23$), CF carrier ($n = 38$), CHT ($n = 35$), or normal NBS ($n = 35$). The parents of children with CF reported higher perceptions of child vulnerability and fathers of children who were CF carriers, viewed their children as more attached. The findings also indicated that infant feeding problems, particularly in the presence of a serious health condition like CF, could represent an important sign of more deeply rooted concerns regarding the parent–child relationship [18].

A study in the UK to explore parents' experience of receiving a positive NBS result used semi-structured interviews with 12 mothers (five with a child with CF and seven with a child with SCD and 10 fathers (five each with a child with CF or SCD) of children diagnosed via NBS [19]. The mothers of infants with a positive NBS for CF found being alone when they received their child's positive CF NBS result upsetting and fathers expressed distress at not being able to support their partner during this time. This also reportedly had the potential to impact on parental relationships as the mother then became responsible for informing the baby's father of the positive CF NBS result. These findings were not reported by the parents of babies who had received a positive NBS for SCD who described being aware of their 'risk' due to the results of antenatal screening [19]. Therefore they were less shocked by the result but were more concerned with the stigma associated with a diagnosis of SCD, which has been commonly cited in the literature [20]. Conversely, the parents of babies with a positive NBS results for CF did not report feeling stigma associated with the condition. CF NBS results also impacted on parental relationships in other ways, including parents questioning their choice of partner and feelings of confusion and guilt at having passed the defective gene on to their child. This was similar to the responses of parents whose baby had received a positive NBS for SCD and perhaps reflects the genetic implications of both conditions.

Receiving the CF NBS result from a health professional perceived to be less informed and therefore unable to answer parental questions about CF was also undesirable and had the potential to impact on future relationships with that health professional [19]. It should be noted that the sample size in this study was small but reflects the findings of other studies. A prospective questionnaire survey of 138 parents who had received a positive CF NBS in Switzerland indicated that most parents ($n = 122$; 88%) were satisfied with screening, four (3%) were not, and 12 (9%) were unsure. The parents received their child's positive CF NBS result over the telephone from a CF physician and were invited for diagnostic testing during the same conversation; 100 (74%) of the parents found the information provided satisfactory. This supports the importance of the person reporting the NBS result having condition specific knowledgeable. The remaining parents who were unsatisfied stated the caller had not explained the test result and the disease or had provided superficial information and instead focused on arranging the appointment [21].

A study in Germany evaluating CF NBS since its introduction in 2016 found that of the 105 (54.7%) families involved in the study (out of 192 who had gone through diagnostic testing after a positive CF NBS result), only 30 parents obtained information about the newborn screening by a physician despite this being mandatory in Germany. Despite this, parents being informed about the positive CF NBS result by a CF specialist were more satisfied with the given information than those informed by the maternity ward. Furthermore, waiting for more than 3 days between the information about the CF NBS result and the diagnostic testing was too long for 77.7% of the families [22]. These findings and those of the study in Switzerland [21] highlight the importance of ensuring that diagnostic testing is undertaken in a timely manner to reduce the parental anxiety and uncertainty associated with the positive NBS result.

Evidence also exists regarding the impact of communicating practices specifically for NBS carrier results. Semi-structured face-to-face interviews conducted with 49 mothers, 16 fathers and 2 grandparents of 51 infants identified CF NBS as carriers of CF ($n = 27$) and SCD ($n = 24$), in England demonstrated untoward anxiety or distress among parents was influenced by how results were conveyed rather than the carrier result per se [23].

In summary, communication of positive CF NBS can influence outcomes in the short term [17,19,21,23] but may also have a longer term impact on children and families [18]. Evidence suggests that the distress caused can manifest in several ways, including arguments between couples, including the apportioning of blame [19,23], the alteration of life plans, an inability to conduct the tasks of daily living, such as going to work or socializing [23], long-term alterations in parent–child relationships [18], and mistrust and lack of confidence affecting ongoing relationships with staff [19].

4. Dealing with Uncertainty: False Positives and CF Screen Positive, Inconclusive Diagnosis (CFSPID)

It has already been highlighted that the time period during which the NBS result is communicated to families but before the confirmatory test results are available, is a "period of maximal uncertainty" [3]. The impact of uncertainty associated with NBS results has been considered extensively in the literature and similar issues have been identified for many of the conditions included in NBS programmes. This is an important consideration that is by no means exclusive to the CF community but may be more prevalent in conditions with a genetic origin such as CF, SCD, and the metabolic conditions due to the longer term implications such as the effect on future reproductive decisions [24–26].

False positive NBS results have the potential to lead to ongoing uncertainty for parents. However, engaging the parents of children who have received a false positive results for any of the conditions included in NBS programmes in research, is notoriously difficult. Studies that have managed to capture this study population have produced conflicting information regarding the potential for false positive results to have a detrimental effect on the family system.

In France, a prospective study conducted with 86 families at 3, 12, and 24 months after receiving a false positive CF NBS result using the Perceived Stress Scale, and the Vulnerable Child Scale found that although 96.5% of parents said they had been anxious at the time of the sweat test, 86% felt entirely reassured 3 months afterwards. The mean perceived stress scale scores did not differ from the French population and the mean vulnerable child scale indicated a low parental perception of child vulnerability. These scores were not found to differ at 12 and 24 months after receiving the false positive CF NBS result. Indeed, 86% to 100% of families no longer worried about CF and all parents stated that they would have the test performed again for another child [27].

Similarly, in the Netherlands, 62 parents (59%) who had received a false positive CF NBS result, and 146 parents (46%) who had received a negative CF NBS result, returned questionnaires to assess long-term effects of false positive results on parental anxiety and stress. In addition, 24 mothers and three fathers participated in 25 semi-structured interviews. Parents showed strong negative feelings after being informed about the positive CF NBS screening result and satisfaction with time of referral was negatively associated with the number of days between being informed and the appointment at the hospital ($r = 0.402$; $p = 0.001$), indicating the importance of timely confirmatory testing. After confirmation that their child was healthy and not affected by CF, most parents felt reassured. Indeed, parental concern about their baby's health or the number of visits to their General Practitioner did not differ significantly between the false positive and the negative NBS groups. After six months, no difference in anxiety levels between both groups of parents was found. Only 6% (4/62) of parents who received a false positive CF NBS result said they would not participate in NBS in the future, while 16% (10/62) were not sure [16].

Likewise, a study in Canada that included 134 mothers who had received a false positive CF NBS for their child and 411 controls who completed questionnaires when their infant was 2 and 12 months old and 54 mothers who had received a false positive CF NBS for their child who were interviewed found that mean anxiety, distress, and vulnerability scores did not differ between the two groups. Of those who received a false positive CF NBS result, 61% were informed by their primary care physician and 39% by a genetic counsellor. The majority (87%) of mothers stated the time between being notified of the positive screen and learning the final results was the "scariest time of their lives", stating that having been home from hospital with an apparently healthy infant, it was alarming to learn that their child might have a chronic illness. Mothers placed tremendous value on the fact that time to confirmatory testing was quick (generally ≤48 h) and valued the excellent coordination of care, particularly being given a time and location to attend for confirmatory testing. Mothers in this study valued the screening system of care in mitigating concerns [28].

Conversely, interviews with 87 parents of 44 infants in the US who had been identified as CF carriers following a false positive CF NBS result found that this resulted in poor intra and interpersonal relationships within the family system and more widely. The parents expressed concerns about test accuracy, the child's health, especially in those who had exhibited signs of respiratory illness, and the future. Parents described the period of uncertainty ending in the child being a carrier rather than being affected by CF, enabling them to gain new perspectives and strengthen their relationship. For one father in the study, the false positive result led to him questioning the child's paternity. The authors also describe extended family members searching for the source of the genetic defect that had led to the child's carrier status; wondering if other relatives had CF and/or were carriers. Parents also talked about their support for NBS and feeling empathy for parents of affected children [29]. Interestingly, this study does not mention the time between parents receiving the NBS results and confirmatory testing, which may have mitigated against these negative outcomes [16,27,28].

The relatively recent new designation of CF Screen Positive, Inconclusive Diagnosis (CFSPID) [30] provides another layer of uncertainty for CF NBS. However, there is very little available evidence about the psychological impact of a CFSPID designation on families. A secondary analysis of interview data obtained from a small subset of five couples when their infants were 2 to 6 months old and later at 12 months of age who participated in a larger project demonstrated that uncertainty emerged as the central dimension of parents' experience when given a CFPSID designation for their child. This uncertainty was linked to the fact that the screening and diagnostic test results were perceived as being contradictory; the presence of two CF mutations from the screening result, usually resulting in an abnormal diagnostic test, CF symptoms, and a CF diagnosis, was confusing to parents, as their child had a normal or borderline sweat test result and were asymptomatic. Moreover, the lack of existing knowledge about the prognostic implications of the identified mutations left health professionals and parents with little certainty about the implications for the infants' future health trajectory [31]. A more recent study with eight parents (three couples and two mothers) supported these initial findings and suggested that CFSPID results caused parental distress, initiated with the first communication of the result and persisting thereafter, but that approaches to the delivery of CFSPID results might reduce the impact [32]. This supports the findings of studies discussed above regarding the importance of the approach used to deliver positive NBS results for other conditions but, perhaps more importantly, the knowledge of the person delivering an uncertain result and their ability to alleviate the parental anxiety associated with this uncertainty [10,19,21,22].

Whilst being confusing for parents, the unknown longer term implications of certain NBS outcomes can also be challenging for health professionals. For instance, borderline CHT results can be challenging to manage to ensure best outcomes for the child in the longer term [33]. Similarly, a Canadian study identified uncertainty associated with the diagnostic as well as the prognostic outcomes for infants with certain metabolic conditions. Health care providers in this study also described transferring some of the uncertainty to parents while involving them in the ongoing monitoring of their child for signs and symptoms that may indicate a more serious prognostic outcome than initially suspected. Finally, the importance of being honest about uncertainty rather than seeing it as a weakness was also viewed as being important by health care providers [34]. These studies highlight the difficulties faced by parents trying to understand the NBS outcomes of uncertain long-term significance as well as the importance of health professionals have adequate knowledge and skills to manage these conditions and parental expectations.

5. Conclusions

The findings of the studies presented above demonstrate the importance of carefully considered information provision to reduce psychological impact when imparting positive CF NBS to parents. The method of delivery of information would seem to be far less important than the knowledge of the person responsible and their ability to answer parents' questions and provide reassurance [19,21–23], particularly if a degree of uncertainty is present, such as with CFSPID results [32]. Despite this, the findings of a recent study found that the CF NBS result is communicated by a range of health professionals internationally and that this may not always be the most appropriate or knowledgeable person but is influenced by many factors, including geographical/logistical, legal, financial and cultural constraints [35]. Additionally, a study in the UK found that specific training for professionals involved in communicating positive NBS results is lacking [36] but is clearly needed to ensure they are adequately prepared to undertake this challenging task. This would also help to meet the suggestions contained within the European guidelines regarding the skills CF team members should possess [12].

Ensuring the most appropriate person communicates a positive CF NBS result is particularly important in cases where there may be a degree of uncertainty, such as for false positive CF NBS results or a CFSPID designation [31,32]. Evidence suggests that good information provision and timely confirmatory testing can mitigate against the long-term psychological distress that has previously been considered to be associated with a false positive CF NBS result [16,27,28].

Funding: This research received no external funding.

Conflicts of Interest: The authors declare no conflict of interest.

References

1. Bush, A. Newborn screening for cystic fibrosis—Benefit or bane? *Paediatr. Respir. Rev.* **2008**, *9*, 301–302. [CrossRef] [PubMed]
2. Castellani, C.; Massie, J.; Sontag, M.; Southern, K.W. Newborn screening for cystic fibrosis. *Lancet Respir. Med.* **2016**, *4*, 653–661. [CrossRef]
3. Castellani, C.; Southern, K.W.; Brownlee, K.; Dankert Roelse, J.; Duff, A.; Farrell, M.; Mehta, A.; Munck, A.; Pollitt, R.; Sermet-Gaudelus, I.; et al. European best practice guidelines for cystic fibrosis neonatal screening. *J. Cyst. Fibros.* **2009**, *8*, 153–173. [CrossRef] [PubMed]
4. Farrell, P.M.; White, T.B.; Derichs, N.; Castellani, C.; Rosenstein, B.J. Cystic Fibrosis Diagnostic Challenges over 4 Decades: Historical Perspectives and Lessons Learned. *J. Pediatr.* **2017**, *181*, S16–S26. [CrossRef]
5. Southern, K.W.; Merelle, M.M.; Dankert-Roelse, J.E.; Nagelkerke, A.D. Newborn screening for cystic fibrosis. *Cochrane Database Syst. Rev.* **2009**, CD001402. [CrossRef]
6. Merelle, M.E.; Huisman, J.; Alderden-van der Vecht, A.; Taat, F.; Bezemer, D.; Griffioen, R.W.; Brinkhorst, G.; Dankert-Roelse, J.E. Early versus late diagnosis: Psychological impact on parents of children with cystic fibrosis. *Pediatrics* **2003**, *111*, 346–350. [CrossRef]
7. Weil, L.G.; Charlton, M.R.; Coppinger, C.; Daniel, Y.; Streetly, A. Sickle cell disease and thalassaemia antenatal screening programme in England over 10 years: A review from 2007/2008 to 2016/2017. *J. Clin. Pathol.* **2020**, *73*, 183–190. [CrossRef]
8. De Boeck, K. Cystic fibrosis in the year 2020: A disease with a new face. *Acta Paediatr.* **2020**. [CrossRef]
9. Grob, R. Is my sick child healthy? Is my healthy child sick? Changing parental experiences of cystic fibrosis in the age of expanded newborn screening. *Soc. Sci. Med.* **2008**, *67*, 1056–1064. [CrossRef]
10. Buchbinder, M.; Timmermans, S. Newborn screening for metabolic disorders: Parental perceptions of the initial communication of results. *Clin. Pediatr.* **2012**, *51*, 739–744. [CrossRef]
11. Farrell, P.M.; White, T.B.; Ren, C.L.; Hempstead, S.E.; Accurso, F.; Derichs, N.; Howenstine, M.; McColley, S.A.; Rock, M.; Rosenfeld, M.; et al. Diagnosis of Cystic Fibrosis: Consensus Guidelines from the Cystic Fibrosis Foundation. *J. Pediatr.* **2017**, *181*, S4–S15. [CrossRef] [PubMed]
12. Castellani, C.; Duff, A.J.A.; Bell, S.C.; Heijerman, H.G.M.; Munck, A.; Ratjen, F.; Sermet-Gaudelus, I.; Southern, K.W.; Barben, J.; Flume, P.A.; et al. ECFS best practice guidelines: The 2018 revision. *J. Cyst. Fibros.* **2018**, *17*, 153–178. [CrossRef] [PubMed]
13. Public Health England. *NHS Newborn Blood Spot Screening Programme: Managing Positive Results from Cystic Fibrosis Screening*; Public Health England: London, UK, 2017; pp. 1–20.
14. Wright, S.J.; Jones, C.; Payne, K.; Dharni, N.; Ulph, F. The Role of Information Provision in Economic Evaluations of Newborn Bloodspot Screening: A Systematic Review. *Appl. Health Econ. Health Policy* **2015**, *13*, 615–626. [CrossRef] [PubMed]
15. Schoen, E.J.; Baker, J.C.; Colby, C.J.; To, T.T. Cost-benefit analysis of universal tandem mass spectrometry for newborn screening. *Pediatrics* **2002**, *110*, 781–786. [CrossRef]
16. Vernooij-van Langen, A.M.; van der Pal, S.M.; Reijntjens, A.J.; Loeber, J.G.; Dompeling, E.; Dankert-Roelse, J.E. Parental knowledge reduces long term anxiety induced by false-positive test results after newborn screening for cystic fibrosis. *Mol. Genet. Metab. Rep.* **2014**, *1*, 334–344. [CrossRef]
17. Salm, A.; Yetter, E.; Tluczek, A. Informing parents about positive newborn screening results: Parents' recommendations. *J. Child Health Care* **2012**, *16*, 367–381. [CrossRef]
18. Tluczek, A.; Clark, R.; McKechnie, A.C.; Brown, R.L. Factors affecting parent-child relationships one year after positive newborn screening for cystic fibrosis or congenital hypothyroidism. *J. Dev. Behav. Pediatr.* **2015**, *36*, 24–34. [CrossRef]
19. Chudleigh, J.; Buckingham, S.; Dignan, J.; O'Driscoll, S.; Johnson, K.; Rees, D.; Wyatt, H.; Metcalfe, A. Parents' Experiences of Receiving the Initial Positive Newborn Screening (NBS) Result for Cystic Fibrosis and Sickle Cell Disease. *J. Genet. Couns.* **2016**, *25*, 1215–1226. [CrossRef]
20. Marsh, V.M.; Kamuya, D.M.; Molyneux, S.S. All her children are born that way': Gendered experiences of stigma in families affected by sickle cell disorder in rural Kenya. *Ethn. Health* **2011**, *16*, 343–359. [CrossRef]
21. Rueegg, C.S.; Barben, J.; Hafen, G.M.; Moeller, A.; Jurca, M.; Fingerhut, R.; Kuehni, C.E.; The Swiss Cystic Fibrosis Screening Group. Newborn screening for cystic fibrosis—The parent perspective. *J. Cyst. Fibros.* **2016**, *15*, 443–451. [CrossRef]

22. Brockow, I.; Nennstiel, U. Parents' experience with positive newborn screening results for cystic fibrosis. *Eur. J. Pediatr.* **2019**, *178*, 803–809. [CrossRef]
23. Ulph, F.; Cullinan, T.; Qureshi, N.; Kai, J. Parents' responses to receiving sickle cell or cystic fibrosis carrier results for their child following newborn screening. *Eur. J. Hum. Genet.* **2015**, *23*, 459–465. [CrossRef]
24. Wilkie, D.J.; Gallo, A.M.; Yao, Y.; Molokie, R.E.; Stahl, C.; Hershberger, P.E.; Zhao, Z.; Suarez, M.L.; Labotka, R.J.; Johnson, B.; et al. Reproductive health choices for young adults with sickle cell disease or trait: Randomized controlled trial immediate posttest effects. *Nurs. Res.* **2013**, *62*, 352–361. [CrossRef]
25. Plumridge, G.; Metcalfe, A.; Coad, J.; Gill, P. The role of support groups in facilitating families in coping with a genetic condition and in discussion of genetic risk information. *Health Expect. Int. J. Public Particip. Health Care Health Policy* **2012**, *15*, 255–266. [CrossRef]
26. The Socio-Psychological Research in Genomics (SPRinG) Collaboration; Eisler, I.; Ellison, M.; Flinter, F.; Grey, J.; Hutchison, S.; Jackson, C.; Longworth, L.; MacLeod, R.; McAllister, M.; et al. Developing an intervention to facilitate family communication about inherited genetic conditions, and training genetic counsellors in its delivery. *Eur. J. Hum. Genet.* **2015**, *24*, 794–802. [CrossRef]
27. Beucher, J.; Leray, E.; Deneuville, E.; Roblin, M.; Pin, I.; Bremont, F.; Turck, D.; Ginies, J.L.; Foucaud, P.; Rault, G.; et al. Psychological effects of false-positive results in cystic fibrosis newborn screening: A two-year follow-up. *J. Pediatr.* **2010**, *156*, 771–776. [CrossRef]
28. Hayeems, R.Z.; Miller, F.A.; Barg, C.J.; Bombard, Y.; Kerr, E.; Tam, K.; Carroll, J.C.; Potter, B.K.; Chakraborty, P.; Davies, C.; et al. Parent Experience with False-Positive Newborn Screening Results for Cystic Fibrosis. *Pediatrics* **2016**, *138*, e20161052. [CrossRef]
29. Tluczek, A.; Orland, K.M.; Cavanagh, L. Psychosocial consequences of false-positive newborn screens for cystic fibrosis. *Qual. Health Res.* **2011**, *21*, 174–186. [CrossRef]
30. Munck, A.; Mayell, S.J.; Winters, V.; Shawcross, A.; Derichs, N.; Parad, R.; Barben, J.; Southern, K.W. Cystic Fibrosis Screen Positive, Inconclusive Diagnosis (CFSPID): A new designation and management recommendations for infants with an inconclusive diagnosis following newborn screening. *J. Cyst. Fibros.* **2015**, *14*, 706–713. [CrossRef]
31. Tluczek, A.; Chevalier McKechnie, A.; Lynam, P.A. When the cystic fibrosis label does not fit: A modified uncertainty theory. *Qual. Health Res.* **2010**, *20*, 209–223. [CrossRef]
32. Johnson, F.; Southern, K.W.; Ulph, F. Psychological Impact on Parents of an Inconclusive Diagnosis Following Newborn Bloodspot Screening. *Int. J. Neonatal Screen.* **2019**, *5*, 23. [CrossRef]
33. Lain, S.J.; Bentley, J.P.; Wiley, V.; Roberts, C.L.; Jack, M.; Wilcken, B.; Nassar, N. Association between borderline neonatal thyroid-stimulating hormone concentrations and educational and developmental outcomes: A population-based record-linkage study. *Lancet Diabetes Endocrinol.* **2016**, *4*, 756–765. [CrossRef]
34. Azzopardi, P.J.; Upshur, R.E.G.; Luca, S.; Venkataramanan, V.; Potter, B.K.; Chakraborty, P.K.; Hayeems, R.Z. Health-care providers' perspectives on uncertainty generated by variant forms of newborn screening targets. *Genet. Med.* **2019**, 1–8. [CrossRef]
35. Chudleigh, J.; Ren, C.L.; Barben, J.; Southern, K.W. International approaches for delivery of positive newborn bloodspot screening results for CF. *J. Cyst. Fibros.* **2019**, *18*, 614–621. [CrossRef]
36. Chudleigh, J.; Chinnery, H.; Bonham, J.R.; Olander, E.K.; Moody, L.; Simpson, A.; Morris, S.; Ulph, F.; Bryon, M.; Southern, K.W. A qualitative exploration of health professionals' experiences of communicating positive newborn bloodspot screening results for nine conditions in England. *BMJ Open* **2020**, in press.

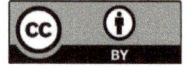

© 2020 by the authors. Licensee MDPI, Basel, Switzerland. This article is an open access article distributed under the terms and conditions of the Creative Commons Attribution (CC BY) license (http://creativecommons.org/licenses/by/4.0/).

MDPI
St. Alban-Anlage 66
4052 Basel
Switzerland
Tel. +41 61 683 77 34
Fax +41 61 302 89 18
www.mdpi.com

International Journal of Neonatal Screening Editorial Office
E-mail: ijns@mdpi.com
www.mdpi.com/journal/ijns

www.ingramcontent.com/pod-product-compliance
Lightning Source LLC
LaVergne TN
LVHW070552100526
838202LV00012B/449